Drugs in Anaesthesia and Intensive Care

THIRD EDITION

MARTIN SASADA

Consultant Anaesthetist
Royal United Hospital
Bath

and

SUSAN SMITH

Consultant Anaesthetist
Cheltenham General Hospital
Cheltenham

OXFORD
UNIVERSITY PRESS

OXFORD
UNIVERSITY PRESS

Great Clarendon Street, Oxford OX2 6DP

Oxford University Press is a department of the University of Oxford.
It furthers the University's objective of excellence in research, scholarship,
and education by publishing worldwide in

Oxford New York

Auckland Cape Town Dar es Salaam Hong Kong Karachi
Kuala Lumpur Madrid Melbourne Mexico City Nairobi
New Delhi Shanghai Taipei Toronto

With offices in

Argentina Austria Brazil Chile Czech Republic France Greece
Guatemala Hungary Italy Japan Poland Portugal Singapore
South Korea Switzerland Thailand Turkey Ukraine Vietnam

Oxford is a registered trade mark of Oxford University Press
in the UK and in certain other countries

Published in the United States
by Oxford University Press Inc., New York

© Oxford University Press 2003

British Library Cataloguing in Publication Data

Data available

Library of Congress Cataloging in Publication Data

Data available

Typeset by Newgen Imaging Systems (P) Ltd., Chennai, India

Printed in Italy by Legoprint S.p.a

ISBN 0 19 852616 4
ISBN 978-0-19-923583-4 Part 1
ISBN 978-0-19-923584-1 Part 2

OXFORD MEDICAL PUBLICATIONS

Drugs in Anaesthesia and Intensive Care

THIRD EDITION

PART 2 : I–Z

Preface to the third edition

This book continues in its original structured format. Advances in pharmacology and medicine have required some rewriting and we hope it continues to be useful for anaesthetists in training, operating department personnel, and for examination purposes. Any comments or criticisms would be gratefully received via email (susan.smith@egnhst.org.uk).

M.P.S.
S.P.S.
March 2003

Preface to the second edition

In this edition we have retained the format of the original; the major changes being the removal of a number of less important or defunct agents. The text for the remainder has been updated to encompass significant developments since 1990.

The first edition proved popular and hopefully useful for preparation for postgraduate examinations in anaesthesia; we trust that this will remain true for the new examinations format.

Cheltenham   M.P.S.
February 1997   S.P.S.

Preface to the first edition

The aim of this book is twofold: firstly to summarise concisely the main pharmacodynamic and pharmacokinetic properties of the drugs with which the practising anaesthetist might be expected to be familiar. Secondly, it seeks to introduce the candidate for the FRCAnaes (and in particular for the second part of this examination) to an ordered scheme for the presentation of information, which we have found to be of value in both the written and oral sections of the examinations. Examiners are more likely to turn a blind eye to minor errors or omissions of knowledge if they are in the context of a clear and well-ordered presentation. A further advantage of this scheme of presentation is that it allows rapid access to specific information. It is our hope that this compendium will prove to be a useful rapid source of reference for clinical anaesthetists in their day-to-day endeavours, both in the theatre and intensive care unit.

This book is intended to complement, rather than to replace, the standard texts on pharmacology for anaesthetists, since it includes no discussion of the principles of pharmacology, an understanding of which is essential for the clinical use of drugs. We feel that these aspects are very satisfactorily covered elsewhere.

Although our research has been as comprehensive as possible, there will obviously remain some information that will have eluded us, or perhaps remains to be discovered. Many practitioners will disagree with our choice of 172 drugs. Any comments or suggestions will be most gratefully and humbly received, in order that further editions of this book may hopefully prove to be more useful.

Finally, we should like to thank the members of the Oxford Regional Drug Information Unit, the many drug company information departments and all our colleagues for their help and support in this venture. In particular, we should like to thank Professor Roy Spector and Drs John Sear and Tim Peto for their invaluable advice on the manuscript.

Oxford
1990

M.P.S.
S.P.S.

Foreword

The ever-increasing size of pharmacological textbooks bears witness to the increased number of drugs on the market and to the greater knowledge of their properties. It is no longer possible for the average doctor to memorise all the information relevant to clinical practice and there is, therefore, a need for a concise handbook which contains the essential information in an easily accessible form.

This book satisfies that need. The authors have been closely concerned with the teaching of pharmacology to junior doctors and have evolved a standardised format for the description of each drug which not only facilitates reference but also aids learning.

They have included most of the drugs commonly used in anaesthesia and intensive care so that the information should prove particularly valuable to junior doctors working in these fields. However, I suspect that this volume will soon become the first source of reference for their senior colleagues as well!

M.K. Sykes
Emeritus Nuffield Professor of Anaesthetics
Oxford, UK

How to use this book

The layout of this book requires some explanation in order for the reader to gain the maximum benefit. The 181 drugs we have included are arranged in alphabetical order to obviate both reference to an index and artificial categorisation of some drugs. Each drug is presented in an identical format and confined to one or two pages under the following headings:

Uses   The main clinical uses are listed.

Chemical   A brief chemical classification is given.

Presentation   The formulation of the commercially available preparations are described.

Main Action   The fundamental pharmacological properties are briefly indicated.

Mode of Action   The mode of action at a cellular or molecular level (where known) is described.

Routes of Administration/Doses   The manufacturer's recommended dose ranges are listed in this section; alternative clinical uses are also mentioned.

Effects   The pharmacodynamic properties are systematically reviewed. Where a drug has no specific or known action on a particular physiological system, the relevant section has been omitted.
The systems described are:
CVS   Cardiovascular system.
RS   Respiratory system.
CNS   Central nervous system.
AS   Alimentary system.
GU   Genito-urinary system.
Metabolic/Other   Metabolic, endocrine and miscellaneous.

Toxicity/Side Effects   The major side effects are listed, with particular reference to the practice of anaesthesia and intensive care.

Kinetics   The available pharmacokinetic data are provided. Quantitative data are not available for all drugs, particularly the long-established ones. Where information on the absorption, distribution, metabolism or excretion is unavailable for a particular drug, the relevant section has been omitted.

Absorption   Details of the absorption and bioavailability are given.

Distribution   This section provides information on the volume of distribution and degree of protein binding of the drug, together, where appropriate, with details of central nervous penetration, transplacental passage etc.

Metabolism The site and route of metabolic transformation and nature and activity of metabolites are described.

Excretion The excretory pathways, clearance and elimination half-life are listed. Although clearances are usually expressed in ml/min/kg, this has not always been possible, due to inadequacies in the original source material.

Special Points This section describes points of relevance to the practice of anaesthesia and intensive care; in particular, significant drug interactions are reviewed.

This standard format offers great advantages; it enables specific questions to be answered very rapidly. For example, the question 'How is fentanyl metabolised?' may be answered simply by locating the drug alphabetically and then consulting the Metabolism section of the text. This principle holds true for all possible permutations of queries.

Glossary of terms used in this book

ADH	Antidiuretic hormone
ARDS	Adult respiratory distress syndrome
ATP	Adenosine triphosphate
AS	Alimentary system
cAMP	Cyclic adenosine monophosphate
CNS	Central nervous system
COX	Cyclo-oxygenase
CSF	Cerebrospinal fluid
CVS	Cardiovascular system
cGMP	Cyclic guanine monophosphate
DNA	Deoxyribonucleic acid
ECG	Electrocardiogram
EEG	Electroencephalogram
ESR	Erythrocyte sedimentation rate
FEV_1	Forced expiratory volume in 1 second
FiO_2	Inspired oxygen concentration
FVC	Forced vital capacity
GABA	Gamma-aminobutyric acid
GU	Genito-urinary
5-HT	5-hydroxytryptamine
INR	International normalised ratio
MAC	Minimum alveolar concentration
MAOI	Monoamine oxidase inhibitor
mRNA	Messenger ribonucleic acid
MRSA	Methicillin-resistant *Staphylococcus aureus*
NMDA	N-methyl-D-aspartate
NSAID	Non-steroidal anti-inflammatory drug
P_aCO_2	Arterial carbon dioxide tension
PEFR	Peak expiratory flow rate
RS	Respiratory system
tRNA	Transfer ribonucleic acid
V_D	Volume of distribution

Drugs in Anaesthesia and Intensive Care

Part 2 : I–Z

Imipenem

Uses Imipenem is a broad spectrum antibiotic used in the treatment of:
1. urinary and respiratory tract infections
2. intra-abdominal sepsis
3. bone and joint infections and
4. bacteraemia.

Chemical A semi-synthetic thienamycin antibiotic presented in a fixed dose combination with cilastatin, a renal peptidase inhibitor which decreases renal metabolism of imipenem to increase the concentration of active circulating imipenem. Cilastatin otherwise has no effect on the bactericidal activity of imipenem.

Presentation In vials containing 500 mg of imipenem monohydrate with 500 mg of cilastatin sodium or twice the quantities of both.

Main Actions Imipenem has a remarkably wide spectrum of activity – the broadest of any currently available. It is active against Gram-positive and Gram-negative aerobes and anaerobes, including most staphylococcal (including MRSA) and streptococcal species, *Pseudomonas aeruginosa*, *Haemophilus influenzae*, *Neisseria gonorrhoeae*, *Escherichia coli*, *Proteus*, *Klebsiella*, *Salmonella* and *Shigella* sp. It is very active against most beta-lactamase-producing bacteria.

Mode of Action Imipenem inhibits cell wall synthesis by binding covalently to penicillin-binding proteins in the bacterial cell membrane and inhibiting transpeptidases involved in cell wall synthesis. Imipenem may have a post-antibiotic effect.

Route of Administration/Doses The drug is administered by intravenous infusion over 20–30 minutes; the adult dose is 1–2 g daily in 3–4 divided doses. The maximum recommended dose is 50 mg/kg/day.

Effects
CVS Hypotension may occur with rapid intravenous injection.

Toxicity/Side Effects Imipenem is usually well tolerated; gastrointestinal upsets (including pseudomembranous colitis), rashes, eosinophilia and abnormalities of liver function tests may occur. Seizures have been reported in up to 2% of patients receiving imipenem. The drug is highly irritant to veins.

Kinetics

Distribution Imipenem is 20% protein-bound in the plasma; the V_D is 0.23–0.31 l/kg.

Metabolism The drug undergoes partial post-excretory metabolism in the renal proximal tubules via dehydropeptidase-1 (a dipeptidase that is inhibited by cilastatin).

Excretion 60–75% of the dose is excreted unchanged in the urine; the drug is non-cumulative in patients with normal renal function. The clearance is 3–3.67 ml/min/kg and the elimination half-life is approximately 1 hour.

Special Points The dosage should be reduced in renal failure; both drugs are removed by haemodialysis.

Imipenem has low endotoxin-releasing potential; the clinical significance of this is unknown.

Imipramine

Uses Imipramine is used for the treatment of:
1. depression and
2. nocturnal enuresis.

Chemical A dibenzazepine derivative.

Presentation As 10/25 mg tablets and a syrup containing 5 mg/ml of imipramine hydrochloride.

Main Action Antidepressant.

Mode of Action Tricyclic antidepressants may potentiate the action of biogenic amines within the central nervous system by preventing their re-uptake at nerve terminals. They also antagonise muscarinic cholinergic, alpha-1 adrenergic and H_1 and H_2 histaminergic receptors.

Route of Administration/Doses The adult oral dose is 25–50 mg 6–8 hourly.

Effects
CVS Imipramine causes postural hypotension as a result of peripheral alpha-adrenergic blockade; a compensatory tachycardia may develop. The tricyclic antidepressants are also negatively inotropic; they also have characteristic effects on ECG morphology, including T-wave flattening and inversion.
RS Imipramine has little effect on respiratory function when normal doses are used.
CNS The predominant effect of the drug is an antidepressant action, which may take several weeks to develop; sedation, weakness and fatigue are also commonly produced.
AS High doses of imipramine increase the gastric emptying time.
Metabolic/Other The drug may produce excessive sweating by an unknown mechanism.

Toxicity/Side Effects Occur in 5% and include palpitations, dysrhythmias, tremor, confusion, mania and hepatic dysfunction. Anticholinergic side effects (blurred vision, dryness of the mouth, constipation and urinary retention) may also occur. Overdose of the drug may result in fits, coma and fatal dysrhythmias.

Kinetics

Absorption The drug is well absorbed when administered orally; the bioavailability is 19–35%.

Distribution Imipramine is 95% protein-bound in the plasma; the V_D is 15–31 l/kg.

Metabolism   The drug is demethylated to an active form, desimipramine; this is inactivated by hydroxylation with subsequent conjugation to glucuronide.

Excretion   The glucuronide conjugates are excreted in the urine. The clearance is 11–19 ml/min/kg and the elimination half-life is 11–25 hours.

Special Points   Scopolamine and the phenothiazines displace tricyclic antidepressants from their binding sites on plasma proteins and thus increase the activity of the latter; barbiturates increase the rate of hepatic metabolism of tricyclic antidepressants and decrease their activity.

Imipramine accentuates the cardiovascular effects of adrenaline; care should be exercised when local anaesthetic agents containing adrenaline are used in patients receiving the drug. Imipramine also increases the likelihood of dysrhythmias occurring during general anaesthesia.

Imipramine is not removed by haemodialysis.

Indometacin

Uses   Indometacin is used in the treatment of:
1. rheumatoid and osteoarthritis
2. gout
3. ankylosing spondylitis
4. acute musculoskeletal disorders
5. dysmenorrhoea and has been used
6. to promote the closure of a patent ductus arteriosus.

Chemical   An indoleacetic acid derivative.

Presentation   As capsules containing 25/50 mg, as slow-release preparations containing 25/50/75 mg, as 100 mg suppositories and as a suspension containing 5 mg/ml of indometacin.

Main Actions   Analgesic, anti-inflammatory and antipyretic.

Mode of Action   Indometacin acts by inhibiting prostaglandin production (by 60–95% according to dose) by causing reversible blockade of the conversion of arachidonic acid to PGG_2, a reaction catalysed by COX. Indometacin does not exhibit COX selectivity.

Routes of Administration/Doses   The adult oral or rectal dose is 50–200 mg/day in divided doses.

Effects
CVS   The drug may cause hypertension, dysrhythmias and salt and water retention leading to the development of peripheral oedema. It promotes the closure of the ductus arteriosus in neonates.
AS   Indometacin causes hyperaemia of the gastric mucosa and may cause ulceration at high doses. Reversible abnormalities of liver function tests may also occur.
GU   Interstitial nephritis leading to an impairment of renal function and hyperkalaemia occurs infrequently.
Metabolic/Other   Indometacin is a more potent anti-inflammatory agent than aspirin or hydrocortisone and a more potent analgesic and antipyretic agent than aspirin in animal models. It also inhibits platelet aggregation and prolongs the bleeding time (which remains within the normal range).

Toxicity/Side Effects   Occur frequently (in 35–50%) – the list of reported side effects is legion. The most common side effects are gastrointestinal and central nervous system disturbances (headache, dizziness and depression). Hypersensitivity reactions and haemopoietic disturbances may also occur.

Kinetics

Absorption   Indometacin is rapidly and well absorbed after oral administration. The bioavailability is 80% via the oral route and 80% when administered rectally.

Distribution   The drug is 99% protein-bound in the plasma, predominantly to albumin. The V_D is 0.5–0.8 l/kg.

Metabolism   Occurs in the liver by demethylation and deacylation with subsequent conjugation to glucuronide. Enterohepatic cycling of the conjugates occurs.

Excretion   One-third is excreted in the faeces and the rest in the urine; 10% of this is excreted unchanged. The clearance is 1–2.5 ml/min/kg and the elimination half-life is 2.6–11.2 hours.

Special Points   The drug should be taken with food or milk to decrease the incidence of gastrointestinal upsets. Indometacin may increase the effect of co-administered oral anticoagulants and sulphonylureas due to displacement from plasma proteins.

The drug is not removed by haemodialysis.

Insulin

Uses Insulin is used in the management of:
1. type I diabetes mellitus
2. diabetic emergencies
3. the peri-operative control of blood sugar concentration
4. hyperkalaemia and
5. to improve glucose utilisation during total parenteral nutrition and
6. in provocation tests for growth hormone.

Chemical A polypeptide hormone. Human insulin is produced commercially by recombinant DNA techniques; bovine insulin differs by three, and porcine insulin by one amino acid from human insulin.

Presentation A wide variety of insulin preparations is available; the standard preparations contain 100 units/ml. The source may be human recombinant, bovine or porcine and each may be modified by the addition of zinc or protamine to retard absorption.

Main Actions Stimulation of carbohydrate metabolism, protein synthesis and lipogenesis.

Mode of Action Insulin binds to and activates a specific membrane-bound receptor; the effects of this may be mediated by alterations in the intracellular concentrations of cyclic nucleotides. Insulin exerts a direct effect on lipoprotein lipase, increases the rate of transcriptional and translational events during protein synthesis and controls membrane polarisation and ion transport by activating Na^+-K^+-ATPase.

Routes of Administration Insulin may be administered intravenously, intramuscularly and subcutaneously in a dose titrated according to the blood sugar estimations. It may be diluted for intravenous infusion in saline/dextrose, but has an improved stability in gelatin solutions. The apparent dose requirement is increased by 20% when bovine or porcine insulin is used in place of human insulin.

Rapidly acting insulins act within 1 hour and have a duration of action of 5–7 hours; slow-acting preparations act within 4 hours and have a duration of action of 18–36 hours.

Effects

Metabolic/Other Insulin has profound effects upon carbohydrate, fat and protein metabolism. The drug increases the rate of diffusion of glucose into all cells, and specifically into hepatocytes by enhancing the activity of glucokinase (which causes the initial phosphorylation of glucose, thereby 'trapping' glucose intracellularly). The drug increases the rate of glycogen synthesis by enhancing the activity of phosphofructokinase (which is involved in glucose phosphorylation) and glycogen synthetase (which polymerises monosaccharides to form glycogen). Insulin simultaneously inhibits glycogenolysis by an action on phosphorylase and inhibits gluconeogenesis. It also facilitates diffusion of glucose into muscle cells.

Insulin causes fat deposition in adipose tissue by increasing the hepatic synthesis of fatty acids; these are utilised within the liver to form triglycerides which are released into the bloodstream; insulin simultaneously activates lipoprotein lipase in adipose tissue which splits triglycerides into fatty acids, enabling them to be absorbed into adipose tissue where they are stored. The drug also inhibits a hormone-sensitive lipase thereby preventing hydrolysis of triglycerides and facilitates glucose transport into fat cells, leading to an increased supply of glycerol which is used in the manufacture of storage triglycerides.

Insulin causes active transport of amino acids into cells, and increases mRNA translation and DNA transcription; in addition, it inhibits the catabolism of proteins.

The drug also causes an increase in the rate of potassium and magnesium transport into cells.

Toxicity/Side Effects   The commonest acute side effect of insulin is hypoglycaemia. Chronic use may be complicated by localised allergic reactions, lipodystrophy and insulin resistance due to antibody formation.

Kinetics

Absorption   Insulin is inactive when administered orally, since it is destroyed by gastrointestinal proteases.

Distribution   The drug exhibits little protein-binding; the V_D is 0.075 l/kg (0.146 l/kg in the diabetic subject).

Metabolism   Insulin is rapidly metabolised in liver, muscle and kidney by glutathione insulin transhydrogenase.

Excretion   The metabolites appear in the urine. The clearance is 33.3 ml/mm/kg (18.5 ml/min/kg in the diabetic subject) and the elimination half-life is 1.6–3.4 minutes (5.3–7.8 minutes in the diabetic subject).

Special Points   The co-administration of steroids, thyroxine, thiazide diuretics and sympathomimetic agents tend to counteract the effects of insulin on carbohydrate metabolism. Many regimes of insulin administration have been described for the peri-operative management of diabetic patients.

Insulin is not removed by dialysis.

Tight blood sugar control in critical illness has been shown to decrease mortality, especially in surgical patients.

Ipratropium

Uses Ipratropium is used in the treatment of asthma and chronic obstructive airways disease.

Chemical A synthetic quaternary ammonium compound which is a derivative of atropine.

Presentation As an isotonic solution of ipratropium bromide containing 0.25 mg/ml for nebulisation or as a metered-dose aerosol delivering 200 μg/dose (18 μg of which is available to the patient).

Main Actions Bronchodilatation.

Mode of Action Ipratropium acts by competitive inhibition of cholinergic receptors on bronchial smooth muscle, thereby blocking the bronchoconstrictor action of vagal efferent impulses. It may also inhibit acetylcholine enhancement of mediator release by blocking cholinergic receptors on the surface of mast cells.

Routes of Administration/Doses The drug is administered by inhalation of a nebulised solution or aerosol in an adult dose of 100–500 μg 6-hourly or 1–2 puffs 6-hourly respectively. The maximum effect is achieved in 1.5–2 hours and lasts 4–6 hours.

Effects
CVS No effect on cardiovascular function is observed after administration by inhalation. When administered intravenously, tachycardia with an increase in blood pressure and cardiac output and a fall in central venous pressure may result.
RS Bronchodilatation is the principal effect of the drug. No effect is seen on the viscosity or volume of secretions or the effectiveness of mucociliary clearance. The oxygen saturation remains unaltered following the administration of ipratropium.
CNS The drug has no effect, since ipratropium is unable to cross the blood–brain barrier.
AS When given orally in large doses, gastric secretion and salivation are decreased by the drug.

Toxicity/Side Effects None of the typical anticholinergic side effects is observed if ipratropium is administered by inhalation. 20–30% of patients receiving the drug experience transient local effects – dryness or unpleasant taste in the mouth. Local deposition of the nebulised drug on the eye may cause mydriasis and difficulty with accommodation.

Kinetics

Absorption The bioavailability of the drug when administered orally is 3–30% and 5% by the inhaled route.

Distribution   The V_D is 0.4 l/kg.

Metabolism   Ipratropium is metabolised to 8 inactive metabolites.

Excretion   Occurs in approximately equal proportions in the urine and faeces. The clearance is 11.8 l/hour and the elimination half-life is 3.2–3.8 hours.

Special Points   Ipratropium is less effective than beta-adrenergic agonists in the treatment of asthma, although its effectiveness in the treatment of bronchitis appears to be equal to that of the beta-adrenergic agonists. An additive effect with the latter drugs is difficult to prove.

Isoflurane

Uses Isoflurane is used:
1. for the induction and maintenance of general anaesthesia and has been used
2. for sedation during intensive care.

Chemical A halogenated methyl ether which is a structural isomer of enflurane.

Presentation As a clear, colourless liquid with a pungent smell. The commercial preparation contains no stabilisers or preservatives; it is non-flammable in normal anesthetic concentrations. The molecular weight of isoflurane is 184.5, the boiling point 48.5 °C and the saturated vapour pressure is 32 kPa at 20 °C. The MAC of isoflurane is 1.15 (0.50 in 70% nitrous oxide), the oil/water solubility coefficient 174 and the blood/gas solubility coefficient 1.4. The drug is readily soluble in rubber; it does not attack metals.

Main Action General anaesthesia (reversible loss of both awareness and recall of noxious stimuli).

Mode of Action The mechanism of general anaesthesia remains to be fully elucidated. General anaesthetics appear to disrupt synaptic transmission (especially in the area of the ventro-basal thalamus). The mechanism may include potentiation of gamma-amino-butyric acid and glycine receptors and antagonism at NMDA receptors. Their mode of action at the molecular level appears to involve expansion of hydrophobic regions in the neuronal membrane, either within the lipid phase or within hydrophobic sites in cell membrane proteins.

Routes of Administration/Dose Isoflurane is administered by inhalation, conventionally via a calibrated vaporiser. The concentration used for the inhalational induction of anaesthesia is 1–4% and for maintenance, 0.5–3%.

Effects
CVS Isoflurane is a mild negative inotrope; it also causes a marked decrease in the systemic vascular resistance and these two effects produce a decrease in mean arterial pressure. Unlike halothane, isoflurane produces a reflex tachycardia. The drug reduces the rate of phase IV depolarisation, increases the threshold potential and prolongs the effective refractory period. Isoflurane causes coronary vasodilation, which in the presence of fixed coronary arterial stenotic lesions, may lead to redistribution of coronary blood flow from the endo- to epicardium ('coronary steal' effect). Isoflurane is not markedly arrhythmogenic and causes little

sensitisation of the myocardium to the effects of circulating catecholamines.

RS Isoflurane is a respiratory depressant, decreasing the tidal volume with little effect on respiratory rate. A slight increase in P_aCO_2 may occur in spontaneously breathing subjects; the drug also decreases the ventilatory response to hypoxia and hypercapnia. Isoflurane is irritant to the respiratory tract and may cause coughing, breath-holding and an increase in bronchial secretions; it also causes bronchodilatation.

CNS The principal effect of isoflurane is general anaesthesia; the drug has little analgesic effect. The drug increases cerebral blood flow when used in normocapnic patients in a concentration exceeding $1 \times MAC$, leading to an increase in intracranial pressure; it also decreases cerebral oxygen consumption. A decrease in skeletal muscle tone results from the use of isoflurane, mediated by an effect on the post-junctional membrane.

AS Hepatic blood flow is well maintained during the administration of isoflurane.

GU The drug reduces the tone of the pregnant uterus.

Toxicity/Side Effects Isoflurane appears to be a trigger agent for the development of malignant hyperthermia (three reported cases). There have been isolated reports of hepatotoxicity associated with the repeated use of isoflurane; nephrotoxicity does not occur with the use of the drug as the fluoride ion concentrations it produces are insignificant.

Kinetics

Absorption The major factors affecting the uptake of volatile anaesthetic agents are solubility, cardiac output and the concentration gradient between the alveoli and venous blood.

Isoflurane is less soluble in blood than is enflurane; alveolar concentration should therefore reach inspired concentration relatively rapidly, resulting in a rapid induction of anaesthesia (although the irritant nature of the drug tends to offset this effect). An increase in the cardiac output increases the rate of alveolar uptake and slows the induction of anaesthesia. The concentration gradient between alveoli and venous blood approaches zero at equilibrium; a large concentration gradient favours the onset of anaesthesia.

Distribution The drug is initially distributed to organs with a high blood flow (the brain, heart, liver and kidney) and later to less well-perfused organs (muscles, fat and bone).

Metabolism 0.2% of an administered dose is slowly metabolised in the liver, principally by oxidation and dehalogenation.

Isoflurane

Excretion Isoflurane is principally exhaled unchanged; 0.2% of an administered dose is excreted in the urine as non-volatile fluorinated compounds.

Special Points Isoflurane potentiates the action of co-administered non-depolarising relaxants. It is suitable for use in epileptic patients.

Isoprenaline

Uses Isoprenaline is used in the treatment of:
1. complete heart block (whilst awaiting transvenous pacing)
2. asthma
3. torsade de pointes and is used to provide
4. inotropic support.

Chemical A synthetic catecholamine.

Presentation As 30 mg tablets and as clear solutions for injection containing 0.02/1 mg/ml of isoprenaline hydrochloride. An aerosol delivering 80/400 µg of isoprenaline sulphate per metered dose is also available.

Main Actions Positive inotropism, positive chronotropism and bronchodilatation.

Mode of Action Isoprenaline is a beta-adrenergic agonist; its actions are mediated by membrane-bound adenylate cyclase and the subsequent formation of cAMP.

Routes of Administration/Doses The initial adult oral dose is 30 mg 8-hourly; the dose may be increased as required to a maximum of 840 mg/day. The aerosol may be used essentially as required. Isoprenaline may also be administered as an infusion, diluted in water or 5% dextrose, at the rate of 0.5–8 µg/min, according to response. The positive chronotropic effect becomes apparent after 20 minutes.

Effects
CVS Isoprenaline is a powerful positive inotrope and chronotrope and thus causes an increase in the cardiac output and systolic blood pressure. The drug causes a decrease in the peripheral vascular resistance (a beta-2 effect); as a result, the diastolic blood pressure tends to decrease. The drug increases automaticity and enhances atrioventricular nodal conduction; it also increases coronary blood flow which tends to offset the increase in myocardial oxygen consumption that it produces.
RS The drug is a potent bronchodilator and increases anatomical dead space and ventilation/perfusion mismatching, which may lead to hypoxia.
CNS Isoprenaline is a central nervous system stimulant.
AS Isoprenaline decreases gastrointestinal tone and motility; the mesenteric blood supply is increased by the drug.
GU The administration of isoprenaline reduces renal blood flow in normotensive subjects, but may increase renal perfusion in shock states. The drug also reduces uterine tone.
Metabolic/Other In common with adrenaline, isoprenaline increases the plasma concentration of free fatty acids and may cause hyperglycaemia. Isoprenaline inhibits antigen-induced histamine release and the formation of Slow-Releasing Substance of Anaphylaxis.

demonstrates dominant theta activity and loss of the alpha rhythm. At high doses, ketamine exhibits local anaesthetic properties.

AS   Post-operative nausea and vomiting are common; salivation is increased following the administration of the drug. Ketamine has no effect on gastrointestinal motility.

GU   Ketamine increases uterine tone.

Metabolic/Other   The levels of circulating adrenaline and noradrenaline are increased following the administration of ketamine. The tone and activity of striated muscle may also increase.

Toxicity   Transient rashes occur in 15% of patients receiving the drug. Emergence delirium, unpleasant dreams and hallucinations are notable complications of the use of ketamine (vi). The hypertonus produced by ketamine may require positioning of the patient prior to induction. Pain on injection (especially intramuscularly) may be alleviated by combination with lignocaine.

Kinetics

Absorption   Ketamine is well absorbed after oral or intramuscular administration; the oral bioavailability is 20%.

Distribution   Ketamine is 20–50% protein-bound in the plasma; the V_D is 3 l/kg. The distribution half-life is 11 minutes; recovery is thus primarily due to redistribution from brain to peripheral tissues.

Metabolism   Ketamine is converted in the liver by N-demethylation and hydroxylation of the cyclohexylamine ring. Some of the metabolites are pharmacologically active.

Excretion   The conjugated metabolites are excreted in the urine. The clearance is 17 ml/kg/min and the elimination half-life is 2.5 hours.

Special Points   Antisialogogue premedication is recommended prior to the use of ketamine. Emergence phenomena are less frequent in the young and elderly. These may be reduced in incidence if the patient is left undisturbed during the recovery period or by premedication with opioid–hyoscine or opioid–hyoscine–droperidol. The incidence of unpleasant dreams is reduced by premedication with lorazepam or diazepam.

Ketamine, in low dose, reduces tourniquet hypertension under general anaesthesia.

Ketamine reduces the requirement for inotropic support in septic patients. In animal models of endotoxic shock, ketamine reduces pulmonary damage by enhancing haemodynamic stability and reducing pulmonary hypertension and extravasation.

Ketamine and thiopentone are pharmaceutically incompatible.

Incidents of abuse have been reported.

Labetalol

Uses Labetalol is used in the treatment of:
1. all grades of hypertension
2. hypertensive emergencies and has been used
3. to produce controlled hypotension during anaesthesia
4. for the control of the reflex cardiovascular responses to intubation and
5. in the management of acute myocardial infarction.

Chemical A synthetic salicylamide derivative.

Presentation As a clear solution for injection containing 5 mg/ml, and as 50/100/200/400 mg tablets of labetalol hydrochloride.

Main Action Antihypertensive.

Mode of Action Labetalol acts by selective antagonism of alpha-1, beta-1 and beta-2 adrenoceptors (the ratio of alpha: beta effects is 1:3 when administered orally and 1:7 when administered intravenously). The drug has some intrinsic sympathomimetic activity at beta-2 adrenoceptors and may cause some vasodilation directly by stimulation of beta-2 receptors in vascular smooth muscle.

Routes of Administration/Doses The adult oral dose is 100–800 mg 12-hourly. The drug may also be administered intravenously as a 5–20 mg bolus injected over 2 minutes, with subsequent increments to a maximum adult dose of 200 mg, or by infusion (diluted in dextrose or dextrose saline) at the rate of 20–160 mg/hour. When administered intravenously, labetalol acts in 5–30 minutes and has a mean duration of action of 50 minutes.

Patients should remain supine whilst receiving the drug via the intravenous route and subsequently assume the upright position cautiously, as profound postural hypotension may occur.

Effects
CVS Intravenous labetalol causes a 20% (greater in hypertensive patients) decrease in the systolic and diastolic blood pressure; the heart rate and cardiac output may decrease by 10%. The drug reduces the systemic vascular resistance by 14%; limb blood flow increases and coronary vascular resistance may decrease. Labetalol inhibits platelet aggregation *in vitro*.
RS With single doses, the drug has no effect on FEV_1, FVC or specific airways resistance in patients with obstructive airways disease. Chronic use of the drug has no clinically significant effect on respiratory function.
CNS Labetalol has no effect on cerebral blood flow; autoregulation is well maintained.

GU   Labetalol decreases renal vascular resistance by 20%, leading to an increase in renal blood flow. The glomerular filtration rate, however, remains unchanged.

Metabolic/Other   The concentrations of adrenaline, noradrenaline and prolactin increase acutely in hypertensive patients given labetalol intravenously. The drug may also decrease plasma renin activity and the concentration of angiotensin II. The ESR and serum transaminase concentration may increase following the administration of the drug; labetalol has no effect on plasma lipid concentration.

Toxicity/Side Effects

The side effects of beta-blockade (asthma, Raynaud's phenomenon, heart failure, cramps, nightmares etc.) occur less frequently during the use of labetalol than do the side effects of alpha-blockade (dizziness, formication, nasal congestion etc.). Gastrointestinal disturbances may also complicate the use of labetalol.

Kinetics

Absorption   Labetalol is rapidly absorbed when administered orally but, due to a significant first-pass metabolism, the bioavailability shows an eight-fold variation (11–86%).

Distribution   The drug is 50% protein-bound in the plasma; the V_D is 2.5–15.7 l/kg.

Metabolism   Labetalol is extensively metabolised in the liver (and possibly in the gut-wall) to several inactive conjugates.

Excretion   Occurs predominantly as inactive conjugates in the urine (5% is excreted unchanged) with some appearing in the faeces. The clearance is 13–31 ml/min/kg) and the elimination half-life is 3–8 hours. Renal impairment has no effect on the kinetics of labetalol; the dose should be reduced in the presence of hepatic impairment.

Special Points   In the presence of concentrations of halothane >3%, labetalol causes a significant decrease in cardiac output, stroke volume, mean arterial pressure and central venous pressure.

Haemodialysis will remove <1% of a dose of labetalol.

Levo thyroxine/ Triiodothyronine

Uses   Thyroid hormones are used in the treatment of:
1. hypothyroidism
2. myxoedema coma and
3. goitre.

Chemical   Both hormones are iodine-containing amino acid derivatives of thyronine.

Presentation   Levo thyroxine is presented as tablets containing 50/100 µg of levo thyroxine sodium. Triiodothyronine is presented as 20 µg tablets and a white lyophilised powder for reconstitution in water containing 20 µg of triiodothyronine.

Main Actions   Modulation of growth and metabolism.

Mode of Action   The thyroid hormones, probably predominantly triiodothyronine, combine with a 'receptor protein' within the cell nucleus and thereby activate the DNA transcription process leading to an increase in the rate of RNA synthesis and a generalised increase in protein synthesis.

Routes of Administration/Doses   The adult oral dose of levo thyroxine is 25–300 µg daily in divided doses, titrated according to the clinical response and results of thyroid function tests. The corresponding dose of triiodothyronine is 10–60 µg daily; the dose by the intravenous route is 5–20 µg 4–12 hourly; close monitoring is essential during intravenous administration. There is a 24-hour latency period before the effects of levo thyroxine are manifested; the peak effect occurs in 6–7 days. Triiodothyronine acts in 6 hours and the peak effect is observed within 24 hours.

Effects
CVS   The thyroid hormones are positively inotropic and chronotropic; these effects may be mediated by an increase in the number of myocardial beta-adrenergic receptors. The systolic blood pressure is increased by 10–20 mmHg; the diastolic blood pressure decreases and mean arterial pressure remains unchanged. Vasodilation results from the increase in peripheral oxygen consumption; the circulating blood volume also increases slightly.
RS   The thyroid hormones increase the rate and depth of respiration secondary to the increase in the basal metabolic rate.
CNS   The hormones have a stimulatory effect on central nervous system function; tremor and hyperreflexia may result. Their physiological function also includes mediation of negative feedback on the release of thyroid-stimulating hormone from the pituitary.

AS Appetite is increased following the administration of levo thyroxine or triiodothyronine; the secretory activity and motility of the gastrointestinal tract are also increased.

GU The thyroid hormones are involved in the control of sexual function and menstruation.

Metabolic/Other Thyroid hormones promote gluconeogenesis and increase the mobilisation of glycogen stores. Lipolysis is stimulated leading to an increase in the concentration of free fatty acids; hypercholesterolaemia may result from increased cholesterol turnover. The rate of protein synthesis is enhanced.

Toxicity/Side Effects Excessive administration of the thyroid hormones results in the clinical state of thyrotoxicosis.

Kinetics

Absorption Both levo thyroxine and triiodothyronine are completely absorbed when administered orally.

Distribution Both hormones are bound to thyroid-binding globulin and thyroid-binding pre-albumin in the plasma; levo thyroxine is 99.97% bound and triiodothyronine is 99.5% bound. The V_D of levo thyroxine is 0.2 l/kg and that of triiodothyronine is 0.5 l/kg.

Metabolism 35% of levo thyroxine is converted to triiodothyronine in the periphery (predominantly in the liver and kidney) and some to inactive reverse T3. Both levo thyroxine and triiodothyronine undergo conjugation to glucuronide and sulphate and are excreted in the bile; some enterohepatic circulation occurs.

Excretion 20–40% of an administered dose is excreted in the faeces unchanged. The clearance of levo thyroxine is 1.7 ml/min and the elimination half-life is 6–7 days; the clearance of triiodothyronine is 17 ml/min and the elimination half-life is 2 days.

Special Points The thyroid hormones increase the anticoagulant activity of co-administered warfarin. Beta-adrenergic antagonists interfere with the conversion of levo thyroxine to triiodothyronine and lead to a relative increase in the inactive reverse T3 fraction.

A 'sick' euthyroid state has been described in critical illness.

Lidocaine

Uses Lidocaine is used:
1. as a local anaesthetic and
2. in the treatment of ventricular dysrhythmias.

Chemical A tertiary amine which is an amide derivative of diethylaminoacetic acid.

Presentation As a clear, colourless 0.5/1/1.5/2% solution for injection of lidocaine hydrochloride (with or without 1:200 000 adrenaline); a gel containing 21.4 mg/ml of lidocaine hydrochloride (with or without chlorhexidine gluconate); a 5% ointment, a 10% spray and a 4% aqueous solution for topical application and as a cream/suppositories (in combination with hydrocortisone) for rectal administration.

Main Actions Reversible neural blockade and class Ib antiarrhythmic actions.

Mode of Action Local anaesthetics diffuse in their uncharged base form through neural sheaths and the axonal membrane to the internal surface of cell membrane sodium ion channels; here they combine with hydrogen ions to form a cationic species which enters the internal opening of the sodium ion channel and combines with a receptor. This produces blockade of the sodium ion channel, thereby decreasing sodium ion conductance and preventing depolarisation of the cell membrane.

Routes of Administration/Doses Lidocaine may be administered topically, by infiltration, intrathecally or epidurally; the toxic dose of lidocaine is 3 mg/kg (7 mg/kg with adrenaline). The adult intravenous dose for the treatment of acute ventricular dysrhythmias is a bolus injection of 1 mg/kg, administered over 2 minutes. This is normally followed by an infusion which begins at the rate of 4 mg/min for the first hour, 2 mg/min for the next hour and subsequently of 1 mg/min. Lidocaine acts in 2–20 minutes, dependent on the rate of administration and has a duration of action of 200–400 minutes (dependent upon the presence of vasoconstrictors and the concentration used).

Effects

CVS In low concentrations, lidocaine decreases the rate of phase IV depolarisation, the duration of the action potential, the effective refractory period and conduction velocity. It has few haemodynamic effects when used in low doses, except to cause a slight increase in the systemic vascular resistance leading to a mild increase in the blood pressure. In toxic concentrations, the drug decreases peripheral vascular resistance and myocardial contractility, producing hypotension and possibly cardiovascular collapse.

RS The drug causes bronchodilatation at subtoxic concentrations. Respiratory depression occurs in the toxic dose range.
CNS The principal effect of lidocaine is reversible neural blockade; this leads to a characteristically biphasic effect in the central nervous system. Initially, excitation (lightheadedness, dizziness, visual and auditory disturbances and fitting) occurs, due to the blockade of inhibitory pathways in the cortex; with increasing doses, depression of both facilitatory and inhibitory pathways occur, leading to central nervous system depression (drowsiness, disorientation and coma). Local anaesthetic agents block neuromuscular transmission when administered intra-arterially; it is thought that a complex of neuro-transmitter, receptor and local anaesthetic is formed which has negligible conductance.
AS Local anaesthetics depress contraction of the intact bowel.
Metabolic/Other Lidocaine may have some anticholinergic and antihistaminergic activity.

Toxicity/Side Effects Allergic reactions to the amide-type local anaesthetic agents are extremely rare. The side effects are predominantly correlated with excessive plasma concentrations of the drug, as described above. Lidocaine has a relatively narrow therapeutic index; its toxicity is related to the cardiac output (and therefore to the hepatic blood flow).

Kinetics

Absorption The absorption of local anaesthetic agents is related to:
1. the site of injection (intercostal > epidural > brachial plexus > subcutaneous)
2. the dose – a linear relationship exists between the total dose and the peak blood concentrations achieved and
3. the presence of vasoconstrictors, which delay absorption.
The bioavailability of lidocaine by the oral route is 24–46%, due to a high extraction and first-pass metabolism by the liver.

Distribution Lidocaine is 64% protein-bound in the plasma, predominantly to alpha-1 acid glycoprotein; the V_D is 0.7–1.5 l/kg.

Metabolism 70% of the dose is metabolised in the liver by N-dealkylation with subsequent hydrolysis to mono-ethyl-glycine and xylidide; the latter is further metabolised prior to excretion in the urine.

Excretion Less than 10% of an administered dose is excreted unchanged in the urine. The clearance is 6.8–11.6 ml/min/kg and the elimination half-life is 90–110 minutes. The clearance is reduced in the presence of cardiac and hepatic failure.

Lidocaine

Special Points The onset and duration of conduction blockade is related to the pKa, lipid solubility and extent of protein binding of the drug. A low pKa and a high lipid solubility are associated with a rapid onset time; a high degree of protein binding is associated with a long duration of action. The pKa of lidocaine is 7.7 and the heptane:buffer partition coefficient is 2.9.

Due to lidocaine's narrow therapeutic index, plasma concentrations of the drug need to be monitored in patients with cardiac and hepatic impairment.

Lidocaine is not removed by haemodialysis.

Intravenous administration of lidocaine decreases nitrous oxide and halothane requirements by 10% and 28%, respectively. Local anaesthetic agents significantly increase the duration of action of both depolarising and non-depolarising relaxants.

EMLA (Eutectic Mixture of Local Anaesthetics) is a white cream used to provide topical anaesthesia prior to venepuncture, and has also been used to provide anaesthesia for split-skin grafting. It contains 2.5% lidocaine and 2.5% prilocaine in an oil–water emulsion. When applied topically under an occlusive dressing, local anaesthesia is achieved after 1–2 hours and lasts for up to 5 hours. The preparation causes temporary blanching and oedema of the skin; detectable methaemoglobinaemia may also occur.

Linezolid

Uses   Linezolid is used in the treatment of:
1. nosocomial and community-acquired pneumonia
2. complex skin and soft tissue infections and
3. MRSA infection.

Chemical   An oxazolidinone.

Presentation   As 600 mg tablets and a solution for intravenous administration containing 2 mg/ml of linelozid.

Main Action   Antibacterial vs. a wide range of Gram-positive organisms, particularly *Enterococcus, Streptococcus* and *Staphylococcal* sp., and Gram-positive anaerobes including *Clostridium perfringens*.

Mode of Action   Linezolid inhibits bacterial protein synthesis by binding specifically to the 505 ribisomal subunit, thereby preventing initiation complex formation.

Routes of Administration/Doses   The adult oral and intravenous dose is 600 mg 12-hourly.

Toxicity/Side Effects   Headache, abnormalities of liver function tests, taste alteration and gastrointestinal disturbances are common. Fertility may be affected reversibly. Skin and bleeding disorders, phlebitis and pancreatitis may also occur.

Kinetics

Absorption   Linezolid is rapidly absorbed after oral administration and has an oral bioavailability approaching 100%.

Distribution   The drug is 31% protein-bound in the plasma; the V_D is 0.64 l/kg.

Metabolism   Linezolid is metabolised by oxidation to two inactive carboxylic acid metabolites.

Elimination   30% is excreted unchanged in the urine, the metabolites are excreted in the urine and faeces. The elimination half-life is 5 hours and the clearance 120 ml/min.

Special Points   Linezolid is a reversible nonselective MAOI. It enhances the effects of ephedrine on the blood pressure.

Lithium

Uses Lithium is used in the treatment of:
1. mania and hypomania and in the prophylaxis of
2. recurrent bipolar depression
3. recurrent affective disorders and
4. as an adjunct in the treatment of chronic pain of non-malignant origin.

Chemical An alkali metal.

Presentation As tablets containing 200/250/400/450 mg of lithium carbonate.

Main Action Antipsychotic.

Mode of Action The precise mode of action of lithium is unknown; it may act by stabilisation of membranes or by alteration of central neurotransmitter function.

Route of Administration/Dose The adult oral dose is 0.4–1.2 g/day; serum levels should be monitored within one week of starting lithium and regularly thereafter, as the drug has a narrow therapeutic index. The therapeutic level is 0.5–1.5 mmol/l.

Effects
CVS Prolonged lithium therapy may lead to reversible ECG changes, especially T-wave depression.
CNS The drug has no effect on central nervous system function in normal subjects, although an increase in muscle tone occurs commonly. Lithium appears to lower the seizure threshold in epileptics.
GU Over one-third of patients receiving lithium develop polyuria and polydipsia due to antagonism of the effects of ADH.
Metabolic/Other With prolonged use of lithium, retention of sodium (secondary to an increase in aldosterone secretion) may occur, as may hypercalcaemia and hypermagnesaemia. The drug has mild insulin-like effects on carbohydrate metabolism.

Toxicity/Side Effects At therapeutic serum levels, disturbances of thyroid function, weight gain, tremor, pretibial oedema and allergic phenomena may occur. Excessive serum concentrations may result in nausea and vomiting, abdominal pain, diarrhoea, ataxia, convulsions, coma, dysrhythmias and death. Nephrogenic diabetes insipidus occurs in 5–20% of patients on long-term lithium treatment.

Kinetics

Absorption The drug is rapidly absorbed when administered orally; the bioavailability is 100%.

Distribution Lithium exhibits no demonstrable protein-binding in the plasma; the V_D is 0.45–1.13 l/kg.

Excretion 95% of a dose of lithium is excreted in the urine; the remainder in sweat. The clearance is 0.24–0.46 ml/min/kg and the elimination half-life is 14–30 hours.

Special Points Renal, cardiac and thyroid function should be monitored regularly during lithium therapy. Co-administration of lithium and diazepam has been reported to lead to hypothermia; the drug may also increase the duration of action of both depolarising and non-depolarising relaxants.

The drug is removed by haemodialysis.

Lorazepam

Uses Lorazepam is used:
1. in the short-term treatment of anxiety
2. as a hypnotic
3. in premedication and
4. for the treatment of status epilepticus.

Chemical A hydroxybenzodiazepine.

Presentation As 1/2.5 mg tablets and as a clear, colourless solution for injection containing 4 mg/ml of lorazepam.

Main Actions
1. hypnosis
2. sedation
3. anxiolysis
4. anterograde amnesia
5. anticonvulsant and
6. muscular relaxation.

Mode of Action Benzodiazepines are thought to act via specific benzodiazepine receptors found at synapses throughout the central nervous system, but concentrated especially in the cortex and mid-brain. Benzodiazepine receptors are closely linked with GABA receptors, and appear to facilitate the activity of the latter. Activated GABA receptors open chloride ion channels which then either hyperpolarise or short-circuit the synaptic membrane.

Routes of Administration/Doses The adult oral or sublingual dose is 1–4 mg/day in divided doses. The intravenous or intramuscular dose is 0.025–0.05 mg/kg; intramuscular injection is painful.

Effects
CVS Lorazepam appears to have no direct cardiac effects.
RS Mild respiratory depression occurs following the administration of the drug, which is of clinical significance only in patients with lung disease.
CNS The drug produces sedation, anterograde amnesia and an anticonvulsant effect.
AS Lorazepam has no effect on basal gastric acid secretion, but decreases pentagastrin-stimulated gastric acid secretion by 25%.
Metabolic/Other Circulating cortisol and glucose levels fall when lorazepam is used in premedication, probably secondarily to its anxiolytic effect.

Toxicity/Side Effects Drowsiness, sedation, confusion and impaired coordination occur in a dose-dependent fashion. Paradoxical stimulation has been reported and occurs more frequently when hyoscine is administered concurrently.

Tolerance and dependence may occur with prolonged use of benzodiazepines; acute withdrawal of benzodiazepines in these circumstances may produce insomnia, anxiety, confusion, psychosis and perceptual disturbances.

Kinetics

Absorption Lorazepam has a bioavailability of 90% when administered by the oral or intramuscular route.

Distribution The drug is 88–92% protein-bound in the plasma; the V_D is 1 l/kg. Lorazepam is less extensively distributed than diazepam and thus has a longer duration of action, despite the shorter elimination half-life of lorazepam.

Metabolism Lorazepam is conjugated directly in the liver to glucuronide to form an inactive water-soluble metabolite.

Excretion 80% of an orally-administered dose appears in the urine as the glucuronide. The clearance is 1 ml/min/kg and the elimination half-life is 8–25 hours – this is unaffected by renal disease.

Special Points The co-administration of cimetidine does not impair the metabolic clearance of lorazepam.

The drug is not removed by haemodialysis.

Magnesium sulphate

Uses Magnesium has been used in the management of:
1. pre-eclampsia and eclampsia
2. hypomagnesaemia associated with malabsorption syndromes (especially chronic alcoholism) and critical illness
3. premature labour (as a tocolytic)
4. acute myocardial infarction
5. torsade de pointes and other ventricular dysrhythmias
6. barium poisoning
7. asthma
8. cerebral oedema
9. spasms occurring with tetanus
10. autonomic hyperreflexia secondary to chronic spinal cord injury and is
11. a component of cardioplegic solutions.

Chemical An inorganic sulphate.

Presentation A clear, colourless solution of magnesium sulphate containing 2.03 mmol/ml of ionic magnesium.

Main Actions Magnesium is an essential co-factor in over 300 enzyme systems. It is also essential for the production of ATP, DNA, RNA and protein function.

Mode of Action The precise mechanism of magnesium's anticonvulsant activity remains unknown; it produces a dose-dependent pre-synaptic inhibition of acetylcholine release at the neuromuscular junction.

Routes of Administration/Doses Magnesium sulphate may be administered intravenously or intramuscularly. A number of dose regimes have been described for the use of magnesium sulphate in the management of pre-eclampsia, e.g. 16 mmol administered intravenously over 20 minutes followed by an infusion of 4–8 mmol/hour. Serum concentrations should be monitored repeatedly and the dose adjusted correspondingly. Loss of deep tendon reflexes is a useful clinical sign of impending toxicity.

Effects
CVS Magnesium acts peripherally to cause vasodilation and may cause hypotension when used in high doses. The drug slows the rate of SA node impulse formation and prolongs SA conduction time, the PR interval and AV nodal effective refractory period. Magnesium attenuates both the vasoconstrictor and arrhythmogenic actions of adrenaline.
RS Magnesium is an effective bronchodilator and attenuates hypoxic pulmonary vasoconstriction.
CNS The drug is a CNS depressant and exhibits anticonvulsant properties. High concentrations inhibit catechol release from adrenergic nerve terminals and the adrenal medulla.

AS Magnesium sulphate acts as an osmotic laxative when administered orally.

GU The drug exerts a renal vasodilator and diuretic effect. It decreases uterine tone and contractility; placental perfusion may increase secondary to a decrease in uterine vascular resistance. Magnesium crosses the placenta and may cause neonatal hypotonia and neonatal depression.

Metabolic/Other Magnesium prolongs the clotting time of whole blood, decreases thromboxane B_2 synthesis and inhibits thrombin-induced platelet aggregation.

Toxicity/Side Effects Minor side effects include warmth, flushing, nausea, headache and dizziness. Dose-related side effects include somnolence, areflexia, AV and intraventricular conduction disorders, progressive muscular weakness and cardiac arrest. The toxic effects can be reversed by the administration of calcium. Intramuscular injection of magnesium sulphate is painful.

Kinetics

Absorption 25–65% of ingested magnesium is absorbed.

Distribution Magnesium is 30% protein-bound in the plasma.

Excretion More than 50% of an exogenous magnesium load is excreted in the urine, even in the presence of significant magnesium deficiency.

Special Points Magnesium enhances the effects of other CNS depressants and neuromuscular blocking agents; 30–50% of the normal dose of non-depolarising relaxants should be used to maintain neuromuscular blockade in the presence of magnesium sulphate. Acute administration of magnesium sulphate prior to the use of suxamethonium appears to prevent potassium release and may reduce the incidence and severity of muscle pains.

Magnesium deficiency is present in 20–65% of patients receiving intensive care.

Mannitol

Uses   Mannitol is used:
1. to reduce the pressure and volume of cerebrospinal fluid
2. to preserve renal function during the peri-operative period in jaundiced patients and in those undergoing major vascular surgery
3. in the short-term management of patients with acute glaucoma
4. for bowel preparation prior to colorectal procedures
5. to initiate a diuresis in transplanted kidneys and
6. in the treatment of rhabdomyolysis.

Chemical   An alcohol, derived from Dahlia tubers.

Presentation   As sterile, pyrogen-free solutions of 10% and 20% mannitol in water; crystallisation may occur at low temperatures.

Main Action   Osmotic diuresis and antioxidant.

Mode of Action   Mannitol is a low-molecular-weight (182 daltons) compound and is thus freely filtered at the glomerulus and not reabsorbed; neither does it cross the intact blood–brain barrier. Its action as a diuretic rests upon the fact that it increases the osmolality of the glomerular filtrate and tubular fluid, increasing urinary volume by an osmotic effect. Mannitol decreases CSF volume and pressure by:
1. decreasing the rate of CSF formation and
2. by withdrawing brain extracellular water across the blood–brain barrier into the plasma; if the barker is disrupted, mannitol passes into the brain extravascular space and is ineffective.

Mannitol also acts as a hydroxyl radical scavenger.

Routes of Administration/Doses   For the reduction of elevated intracranial pressure, a dose of 1 g/kg is infused intravenously over 15 minutes prior to operative treatment. Subsequently, intermittent doses of 0.25–0.5 g/kg may be used for the treatment of persistently elevated intracranial pressure. The diuretic dose is 0.5–1 g/kg. Mannitol acts within a few minutes and lasts 1–4 hours.

The oral dose for bowel preparation is 100 ml of the 20% solution – care should be taken to maintain adequate hydration.

Effects
CVS   The acute administration of mannitol increases the cardiac output; blood pressure increases by 5–10 mmHg.
CNS   Mannitol induces a significant reduction in intracranial pressure with preservation of cerebral blood flow in patients with intact autoregulation; in patients with defective autoregulation,

a minimal reduction in intracranial pressure with an increase in cerebral blood flow occurs.

GU Renal blood flow is increased and the rate of renin secretion decreases; mannitol washes out the medullary interstitial gradient, leading to a decreased ability to produce concentrated urine. Diuresis occurs 1–3 hours after administration.

Metabolic/Other The plasma sodium and potassium concentrations may fall and urea increase with the use of high doses of mannitol.

Toxicity/Side Effects Circulatory overload and rebound increases in intracranial pressure may occur following the use of mannitol. Allergic responses are rare; the drug is irritant to tissues and veins. Mannitol may have toxic effects on distal convoluted tubule and collecting duct cells, causing vacuolisation.

Kinetics

Absorption After oral administration, approximately 17.5% is absorbed in the small bowel.

Distribution The drug shows a biphasic distribution to plasma and extracellular water; complex fluid shifts occur in response to this. The V_D is 0.47 l/kg.

Metabolism Mannitol is not metabolised in man.

Excretion The drug is excreted unchanged in the urine: the clearance is 7 ml/min/kg and the elimination half-life is 72 minutes.

Special Points Blood should not be co-administered with mannitol. A total dose exceeding 3 g/kg/day may produce a serum osmolality greater than 320 mOsm/l. Rebound increases in intracranial pressure may occur after the cessation of mannitol therapy.

Metaraminol

Uses Metaraminol is used as an adjunct in the treatment of:
1. hypotension occurring during general or spinal anaesthesia and
2. for the management of hypotension occurring during cardiopulmonary bypass.

Chemical A synthetic sympathomimetic amine.

Presentation As a clear solution containing 10 mg/ml of metaraminol tartrate.

Main Action Peripheral vasoconstriction.

Mode of Action Metaraminol is a direct- and indirect-acting sympathomimetic agent that has agonist effects at both alpha- and beta-adrenoceptors, although alpha-agonist activity predominates.

Routes of Administration/Doses The adult dose by intravenous infusion of metaraminol diluted in saline or dextrose should be titrated according to response; bolus doses of 0.5–5 mg may be administered intravenously with extreme caution. The corresponding intramuscular or subcutaneous dose for the prevention of hypotension is 2–10 mg. The onset of effect after intravenous administration occurs within 1–2 minutes with maximum effect at 10 minutes and lasts 20–60 minutes.

Effects
CVS Metaraminol causes a sustained increase in the systolic and diastolic blood pressure due to an increase in the systemic vascular resistance; it also increases pulmonary vascular resistance. A reflex bradycardia occurs; the drug has positive inotropic properties and the cardiac output may decrease or remain unchanged in normal subjects. The coronary blood flow is increased by metaraminol by an indirect mechanism.
RS The drug causes a slight decrease in the respiratory rate and an increase in the tidal volume.
CNS The cerebral blood flow is decreased by the administration of metaraminol.
GU The renal blood flow is decreased by metaraminol. The drug causes contraction of the pregnant uterus.
Metabolic/Other Metaraminol increases glycogenolysis and inhibits insulin release leading to hyperglycaemia. Lipolysis is similarly increased. The drug may also increase oxygen consumption and body temperature.

Toxicity/Side Effects Headaches, dizziness, tremor and nausea and vomiting may occur with the use of the drug. Rapid and large increases in blood pressure resulting in left ventricular failure and cardiac arrest have been reported after the administration of metaraminol. Extravascular injection of the drug may lead to tissue necrosis and abscess formation at the injection site.

Kinetics There are no quantitative data available.

Metformin

Uses   Metformin is used in the treatment of non-insulin-dependent (type II) diabetes mellitus.

Chemical   A biguanide.

Presentation   As 500/850 mg tablets of metformin hydrochloride.

Main Action   Hypoglycaemia.

Mode of Action   Biguanides have no effect in the absence of circulating insulin; they do not alter insulin concentration but do enhance its peripheral action. They appear to act by inhibiting the intestinal absorption of glucose and decreasing the peripheral utilisation of glucose, both by increasing the rate of anaerobic glycolysis and by decreasing the rate of gluconeogenesis.

Route of Administration/Dose   The adult oral dose is 1.5–3 g daily, in divided doses. Metformin has a duration of action of 8–12 hours.

Effects
AS   Metformin reduces the intestinal absorption of glucose, folate and vitamin B_{12}; it has no effects on gastric motility. The drug may also increase the intestinal utilisation of glucose and cause weight loss.
Metabolic/Other   Metformin increases the sensitivity to the peripheral actions of insulin by increasing the number of low-affinity binding sites for insulin in red blood cells, adipocytes, hepatocytes and skeletal muscle cells. The drug does not cause hypoglycaemia in diabetic subjects receiving metformin monotherapy. Metformin inhibits the metabolism of lactate and causes a decrease in the plasma triglyceride, cholesterol and prebeta-lipoprotein concentrations.

Toxicity/Side Effects   Metformin is normally well tolerated; gastrointestinal disturbances may occur. Lactic acidosis may complicate the use of the drug rarely.

Kinetics

Absorption   The drug is slowly absorbed from the small intestine; the oral bioavailability is 50–60%.

Distribution   Metformin is not protein-bound, in the plasma.

Metabolism   No metabolites of the drug have been detected in man.

Excretion The drug is excreted essentially unchanged in the urine. The clearance exceeds the glomerular filtration rate, implying active tubular secretion. The elimination half-life is 1.7–4.5 hours. The drug is not recommended for use in patients with renal impairment.

Methohexitone

Uses   Methohexitone is used for the induction and maintenance of anaesthesia.

Chemical   A methylated oxybarbiturate.

Presentation   As a white crystalline powder in vials containing 0.1/0.5 g of methohexitone sodium mixed with sodium carbonate; this is dissolved in water before administration to yield a clear, colourless solution with a pH of 11 and a pKa of 7.9 which is stable in solution for 6 weeks.

Main Action   Hypnotic.

Mode of Action   Barbiturates are thought to act primarily at synapses by depressing post-synaptic sensitivity to neurotransmitters and by impairing pre-synaptic neurotransmitter release. Multi-synaptic pathways are depressed preferentially; the reticutar activating system is particularly sensitive to the depressant effects of barbiturates. The action of barbiturates at the molecular level is unknown. They may act in a manner analogous to that of local anaesthetic agents by entering cell membranes in the unionised form, subsequently becoming ionised and exerting a membrane-stabilising effect by decreasing sodium and potassium ion conductance, decreasing the amplitude of the action potential and slowing the rate of conduction in excitable tissue. In high concentrations, barbiturates depress the enzymes involved in glucose oxidation, inhibit the formation of ATP and depress calcium-dependent action potentials. They also inhibit calcium-dependent neurotransmitter release and enhance chloride ion conductance in the absence of GABA.

Routes of Administration/Doses   The drug is usually administered intravenously in a dose of 1–1.5 mg/kg; it acts in one arm–brain circulation time and awakening occurs in 2–3 minutes. The drug may also be administered intramuscularly in a dose of 6.6 mg/kg or rectally in a dose of 15–20 mg/kg.

Effects
CVS   Methohexitone has negatively inotropic effects and decreases systemic vascular resistance; it may also depress transmission in autonomic ganglia and thus lead to hypotension.
RS   Methohexitone is a more powerful respiratory depressant than thiopentone and obtunds the ventilatory response to both hypoxia and hypercarbia. The drug may cause pronounced coughing and hiccuping.
CNS   At low doses, methohexitone may cause paradoxical excitement. Induction of anaesthesia with the drug is associated with an increased incidence of excitatory phenomena

when compared to thiopentone. Methohexitone decreases both the cerebral blood flow and intracranial pressure. The drug may cause epileptiform EEG patterns; abnormal muscle movements may also occur due to neurotransmitter release.

AS The drug causes some depression of intestinal activity and constriction of the splanchnic vasculature.

GU Methohexitone decreases renal plasma flow and increases ADH secretion, leading to a decrease in urine output. It has no effect on the tone of the gravid uterus.

Metabolic/Other The drug decreases the production of superoxide anions by polymorphonuclear leucocytes.

Toxicity/Side Effects Methohexitone causes pain on injection in up to 80% of patients. It is less irritant than thiopentone when extravasation occurs, but when administered intra-arterially may lead to arterial constriction and thrombosis. Anaphylactoid reactions occur with a frequency similar to that observed with thiopentone. Nausea and vomiting may complicate the use of methohexitone.

Kinetics

Distribution The drug is 51–65% protein-bound in the plasma, predominantly to albumin; 20% is sequestered in red blood cells; the V_D is 1.13 l/kg. The rapid onset of action of the drug is due to:

1. the high blood flow to the brain
2. the lipophilicity of the drug and
3. its low degree of ionisation – only the non-ionised fraction crosses the blood–brain barrier (methohexitone is 75% non-ionised at pH 7.4: hyperventilation increases the non-bound fraction and increases the anaesthetic effect). The relatively brief duration of anaesthesia following a bolus of methohexitone is due to redistribution to muscle and later to fat. Methohexitone has a shorter duration of action than thiopentone due to its very short distribution half-life and a high clearance, which is four times greater than that of thiopentone.

Metabolism Occurs in the liver, primarily to a 4-hydroxymetabolite.

Excretion The metabolites are excreted in the urine, < 1% of the dose is excreted unchanged. The clearance is 7.9–13.9 ml/min/kg and the elimination half-life is 1.8–6 hours.

Special Points The drug may induce acute clinical and biochemical manifestations in patients with porphyria and is also not recommended for use in epileptics. Methohexitone should be used with caution in patients with fixed cardiac output states, hepatic or renal dysfunction, myxoedema, dystrophia myotonica, myasthenia gravis, familial periodic paralysis, and in the elderly or in patients who are hypovolaemic.

Methoxamine

Uses Methoxamine is used for:
1. the correction or prevention of hypotension during spinal or general anaesthesia and cardiopulmonary bypass and
2. the treatment of supraventricular tachycardias.

Chemical A synthetic sympathomimetic amine.

Presentation As a clear solution containing 20 mg/ml of methoxamine hydrochloride.

Main Actions Peripheral vasoconstriction and bradycardia.

Mode of Action Methoxamine is a selective alpha-1 adrenergic agonist.

Routes of Administration/Doses Methoxamine is administered intravenously at a rate of 1 mg/min to a total dose of 5–10 mg in an adult; it acts within 1–2 minutes and has a duration of action of 1 hour. The corresponding intramuscular dose is 5–20 mg when the onset of action is 15–20 minutes and duration of effect is 90 minutes.

Effects
CVS Methoxamine commonly produces a reflex and intrinsic bradycardia, accompanied by an increase in the systolic and diastolic blood pressure and central venous pressure. The drug has no effect on the cardiac output, but prolongs the effective refractory period and slows atrio-ventricular conduction.
RS The drug has no effect on respiratory function.
AS Contraction of gastrointestinal sphincters follows the administration of methoxamine.
GU The drug produces renal arterial vasoconstriction leading to a fall in the glomerular filtration rate. Contraction of the pregnant uterus and a decrease in uterine blood flow may occur.
Metabolic/Other Mydriasis, piloerection and diaphoresis are produced by the drug. Glycogenolysis and gluconeogenesis are stimulated; this is accompanied by a decrease in insulin secretion.

Toxicity/Side Effects Headaches, projectile vomiting, sensations of coldness and the desire to urinate have been reported in association with the use of methoxamine.

Kinetics There are no data available.

Special Points The drug may precipitate severe hypertension in patients with uncontrolled hyperthyroidism or who are receiving monoamine oxidase inhibitors or tricyclic antidepressants.

Methyldopa

Uses Methyldopa is used in the treatment of:
1. hypertension and
2. pre-eclampsia.

Chemical A phenylalanine derivative.

Presentation As 125/250/500 mg tablets and a suspension containing 50 mg/ml of methyldopa. A solution for intravenous administration containing 50 mg/ml of methyldopa hydrochloride is also available.

Main Actions Antihypertensive.

Mode of Action Methyldopa is metabolised to alpha-methyl noradrenaline which is stored in adrenergic nerve terminals within the central nervous system; the latter is a potent agonist at alpha-2 (pre-synaptic) nerve terminals and reduces central sympathetic discharge, thereby lowering the blood pressure (cf. clonidine).

Routes of Administration/Dose The adult oral dose is 0.5–3 g/day in 2–3 divided doses.

Effects
CVS Methyldopa decreases the systemic vascular resistance with little accompanying change in either cardiac output or heart rate. Postural hypotension occurs uncommonly with the use of the drug.
GU Methyldopa has little effect on the renal or uteroplacental blood flow, the glomerular filtration rate or filtration fraction.
Metabolic/Other Plasma renin activity and noradrenaline concentrations decrease after administration of the drug.

Toxicity/Side Effects The reported side effects after the administration of methyldopa are legion. Cardiovascular disturbances that may result from the use of the drug include orthostatic hypotension, bradycardia and peripheral oedema. Central nervous system disturbances may also occur, including sedation, depression, weakness, paraesthesiae and dizziness. Gastrointestinal, dermatological and haematological disturbances, including thrombocytopenia, a positive Coomb's test (in 10—20%) and haemolytic anaemia have also been reported. Methyldopa may also cause hepatic damage.

Kinetics

Absorption Methyldopa has a variable absorption when administered orally; the bioavailability is 8–62% by this route, due to a significant first-pass metabolism.

Distribution The drug is 50% protein-bound in the plasma; the V_D is 0.21–0.37 l/kg.

Metabolism Methyldopa is conjugated to sulphate as it traverses the intestinal mucosa, and is metabolised in the liver to a variety of poorly characterised metabolites.

Excretion 20–40% of an administered dose is excreted in the urine; two-thirds of this unchanged. The clearance is 2.2–4 ml/min/kg and the elimination half-life is 2.1–2.8 hours.

Special Points The hypotension effects of the drug are additive with those produced by volatile anaesthetic agents; methyldopa also decreases the apparent MAC of the latter.

The action of the drug is prolonged in the presence of renal failure; it is removed by haemodialysis.

Methyldopa commonly produces nasal congestion; care should be exercised during nasal intubation in patients receiving the drug.

Methylphenidate

Uses   Methylphenidate is used for the treatment of:
1. attention-deficit/hyperactivity disorder (ADHD)
2. narcolepsy and has been used for the treatment of
3. post-anaesthetic shivering
4. hiccuping during general anaesthesia
5. depression and
6. brain injury.

Chemical   A piperidine derivative.

Presentation   As 5/10/20 mg tablets of methylphenidate hydrochloride.

Main Actions   Central nervous stimulation.

Mode of Action   Methylphenidate binds to the dopamine transporter in pre-synaptic cell membranes, blocking its re-uptake, thereby increasing extracellular dopamine levels. It also affects norepinephrine re-uptake and binds weakly to 5HT receptors.

Routes of Administration/Doses   The drug is administered orally, to a maximum of 60 mg/day in divided doses.

Effects
CVS   The drug causes dose-dependent hypertension and tachycardia.
CNS   Methylphenidate causes generalised CNS stimulation.
Endocrine/Metabolic   Methylphenidate decreases growth velocity.

Toxicity/Side Effects   Insomnia, nervousness, anorexia, hypertension and tachycardia occur relatively frequently. The drug has significant potential for abuse.

Kinetics

Absorption   Methylphenidate is almost completely absorbed after oral administration.

Distribution   The drug exhibits a low degree of protein binding.

Metabolism   Occurs primarily to deesterification to ritalinic acid.

Excretion   60–80% of the dose is administered in the urine. The elimination half-life is 2.5 hours.

Metoclopramide

Uses   Metoclopramide is used in the treatment of:
1. digestive disorders, e.g. hiatus hernia, reflux oesophagitis and gastritis
2. nausea and vomiting due to a variety of causes, e.g. drugs (general anaesthetic agents, opiates and cytotoxic gents), radiotherapy, hepatic and biliary disorders
3. diagnostic radiology of the gastrointestinal tract
4. migraine and
5. post-operative gastric hypotonia.

Chemical   A chlorinated procainamide derivative.

Presentation   As 10 mg tablets, 15 mg slow-release capsules, a syrup containing 1 mg/ml and as a clear, colourless solution for injection containing 5 mg/ml of metoclopramide hydrochloride.

Main Actions   Increased gastrointestinal motility and antiemetic.

Mode of Action   The effects of metoclopramide on gastrointestinal motility appear to be mediated by:
1. antagonism of peripheral dopaminergic (D_2-) receptors
2. augmentation of peripheral cholinergic responses and
3. a direct action on smooth muscle to increase tone.

The antiemetic effects of the drug appear to be mediated by:
1. central dopaminergic (D_2-) blockade leading to an increased threshold for vomiting at the chemoreceptor trigger zone and
2. a decrease in the sensitivity of visceral nerves supplying afferent information to the vomiting centre.

Routes of Administration/Doses   Metoclopramide may be administered orally, intravenously or intramuscularly; the adult does by all routes is 10 mg 8-hourly. A dose of 1–2 mg/kg is recommended for the treatment of nausea and vomiting associated with cisplatin treatment.

Effects

CVS   There have been occasional reports of hypotension during general anaesthesia and cardiac arrest, dysrhythmias and hypertension in patients with phaeochromocytoma following the administration of metoclopramide.

CNS   Metoclopramide raises the threshold for vomiting at the chemoreceptor trigger zone and prevents apomorphine-induced vomiting in man. The drug has neuroleptic effects (including an antipsychotic action) as would be expected of a centrally-acting dopamine antagonist.

AS   Metoclopramide increases the tone of the lower oesophageal sphincter by about 17 mmHg, accelerates gastric

emptying and the amplitude of gastric contractions, and accelerates small intestinal transit time. Its effects on large bowel motility are variable. The drug has no effect on gastric secretion.
GU The drug may increase ureteric peristaltic activity.
Metabolic/Other Metoclopramide stimulates prolactin release and also causes a transient increase in aldosterone secretion.

Toxicity/Side Effects Occur in 11% of patients receiving the drug; drowsiness, dizziness, faintness and bowel disturbances are the most frequently reported side effects. Extrapyramidal side effects occur, the most common manifestations are akathisia and oculogyric crises; extrapyramidal effects occur more frequently with higher doses, in patients with renal impairment and in the elderly. The neuroleptic malignant syndrome has been reported in association with metoclopramide.

Kinetics

Absorption The drug is rapidly absorbed after oral administration and has a bioavailability by this route of 32–97%. This wide variability is due primarily to first-pass conjugation to sulphate.

Distribution Metoclopramide is 13–22% protein bound in the plasma; the V_D is 2.2–3.4 l/kg.

Metabolism Occurs primarily in the liver; the major metabolite is a sulphate derivative. Two other metabolites have been identified in man.

Excretion 80% of an oral dose is excreted in the urine within 24 hours; 20% of this is unchanged and the remainder appears as non-metabolised drug conjugated to a sulphate or glucuronide and as the sulphated metabolite. The clearance is 8.8–11.6 ml/min/kg and the elimination half-life is 2.6–5 hours.
  Metoclopramide is not significantly removed by haemodialysis.

Metronidazole

Uses Metronidazole is used for:
1. the treatment and prophylaxis of infections due to anaerobic bacteria, especially *Bacteroides fragilis* and *Clostridia* sp., and the treatment of
2. protozoal infections such as amoebiasis, giardiasis and trichomoniasis
3. acute dental infections and
4. pseudomembranous colitis.

Chemical A synthetic imidazole derivative.

Presentation As 200/400/500 mg tablets; 500 mg or 1 g suppositories and as a clear, colourless, 0.5% solution for intravenous injection of metronidazole.

Main Actions Metronidazole is an antimicrobial agent with a high degree of activity against anaerobes and protozoa.

Mode of Action The drug acts via a reactive intermediate which reacts with bacterial DNA so that the resultant DNA complex can no longer function as an effective primer for DNA and RNA polymerases – all nucleic acid synthesis is thus effectively terminated.

Routes of Administration/Doses The adult oral dose is 200–800 mg, and the corresponding rectal dose is 1 g 8-hourly. The intravenous dose is 500 mg 8-hourly, administered at a rate of 5 ml/min.

Effects
Metabolic/Other Metronidazole decreases the cholesterol content of bile.

Toxicity/Side Effects Unpleasant taste, nausea and vomiting, gastrointestinal disturbances, rashes and darkening of urine have been reported. Peripheral neuropathy and leucopenia may occur with chronic use of the drug.

Kinetics

Absorption The bioavailability of oral metronidazole is 80%, and by the rectal route is 75%.

Distribution Metronidazole is distributed in virtually all tissues and body fluids in concentrations that do not differ markedly from their serum levels. Approximately 10% is protein-bound in the plasma. The V_D is 0.75 l/kg.

Metabolism Occurs by oxidation and glucuronidation in the liver.

Excretion   60% of the dose is excreted unchanged in the urine; the drug does not usually accumulate in renal failure. The clearance is 1.22 ml/kg/min and the elimination half-life is 6–10 hours.

Special Points   Metronidazole increases the anticoagulant effect of warfarin and exhibits a disulfiram-like interaction with alcohol producing an acute confusional state.

Prolongation of the action of vecuronium by the co-administration of the drug has been demonstrated in animals.

Metronidazole may cause reddish-brown discoloration of the urine.

Metronidazole is removed by haemodialysis.

Midazolam

Uses Midazolam is used:
1. for induction of anaesthesia
2. for sedation during endoscopy and procedures performed under local anaesthesia and during intensive care
3. as a hypnotic
4. for premedication prior to general anaesthesia and may be of use
5. in the treatment of chronic pain, including deafferentation syndromes.

Chemical A water-soluble imidazobenzodiazepine.

Presentation As a clear, colourless solution of midazolam hydrochloride containing 1/2/5 mg/ml.

Main Actions
1. hypnosis
2. sedation
3. anxiolysis
4. anterograde amnesia
5. anticonvulsant and
6. muscular relaxation.

Mode of Action Benzodiazepines are thought to act via specific benzodiazepine receptors found at synapses throughout the central nervous system, but concentrated especially in the cortex and mid-brain. Benzodiazepine receptors are closely linked with GABA receptors, and appear to facilitate the activity of the latter. Activated GABA receptors.open chloride ion channels which then either hyperpolarise or short-circuit the synaptic membrane. Midazolam has kappa-opioid against activity *in vitro*, which may explain the mechanism of benzodiazepine-induced spinal analgesia.

Routes of Administration/Doses The intramuscular dose (used for premedication) is 0.07–0.08 mg/kg; the intravenous dose for sedation is 0.07–0.1 mg/kg, titrated according to response. The end point for sedation is drowsiness and slurring of speech – response to commands is, however, maintained. The drug may also be administered intrathecally in an adult dose of 0.3–2 mg or epidurally in a dose of 0.1–0.2 mg/kg.

Effects
CVS Systolic blood pressure decreases by 5% and diastolic pressure by 10% and the systemic vascular resistance falls by 15–33% following the administration of the drug; the heart rate increases by 18%. Midazolam in combination with fentanyl obtunds the pressor response to intubation to a greater extent than thiopentone in combination with fentanyl.

RS Midazolam decreases the tidal volume but this is offset by an increase in the respiratory rare; the minute volume is thus little changed. Apnoea occurs in 10–77% of patients when midazolam is used as an induction agent. The drug impairs the ventilatory response to hypercapnia.

CNS The drug produces hypnosis, sedation and anterograde amnesia. There have been no studies of the anticonvulsant activity of midazolam in man. The cerebral oxygen consumption and cerebral blood flow are decreased in a dose-related manner, but a normal relationship is maintained between the two. When administered intrathecally or epidurally, the drug has antinociceptive effects.

AS A midazolam fentanyl induction sequence is associated with a lower incidence of post-operative vomiting than with a thiopentone fentanyl sequence. The drug reduces hepatic blood flow.

GU Midazolam decreases renal blood flow.

Metabolic/Other Midazolam decreases the adrenergic but not the cortisol and renin response to stress. The drug causes significant inhibition of phagocytosis and leucocyte bactericidal activity.

Toxicity/Side Effects Side effects are confined to occasional discomfort at the site of injection. Withdrawal phenomena may occur in children after prolonged infusion.

Kinetics

Absorption The bioavailability when administered by the oral route is 44% and by the intramuscular route is 80–100%.

Distribution The drug is 96% protein-bound in the plasma; the V_D is 0.8–1.5 l/kg. The V_D may increase to 3.1 l/kg in the critically ill.

Metabolism Midazolam is virtually completely metabolised in the liver to hydroxylated derivatives which are then conjugated to a glucuronide. Metabolites bind to CNS benzodiazepine receptors and are pharmacologically active.

Excretion Occurs in the urine, predominantly as the hydroxylated derivatives; renal impairment thus has little effect. The clearance is 5.8–9 ml/min/kg and the elimination half-life is 1.5–3.5 hours. The elimination half-life may increase to 5.4 hours in the critically ill.

Special Points The short duration of action of midazolam is due to its high lipophilicity, high metabolic clearance and rapid rate of elimination. However, this may not be the case after prolonged dosing on intensive care.

The use of midazolam in premedication decreases the MAC of volatile agents by approximately 15%.

The clinical effects of the drug can be reversed by physostigmine, glycopyrronium and flumazenil.

Mivacurium

Uses Mivacurium is used to facilitate intubation and controlled ventilation.

Chemical A benzylisoquinolinium which is a mixture of three stereoisomers; *trans-trans* (57%), *cis-trans* (36%) and *cis-cis* (4–8%). The *cis-cis* isomer is estimated to have one-tenth of the neuromuscular blocking potency of the other two stereoisomers.

Presentation As a clear, pale-yellow aqueous solution in 5 and 10 ml ampoules containing 2 mg/ml of mivacurium chloride.

Main Action Competitive neuromuscular blockade.

Mode of Action Mivacurium acts by competitive antagonism of acetylcholine at nicotinic (N2) receptors at the postsynaptic membrane of the neuromuscular junction.

Route of Administration/Doses Mivacurium is administered intravenously; the normal intubating dose is 0.07–0.15 mg/kg (0.1–0.2 mg/kg for children aged 2–12 years). Maintenance doses of 0.1 mg/kg are required at approximately 15-minute intervals. The drug may also be infused at a rate of 360–420 µg/hour (600–1000 µg/hour for children aged 2–12). Satisfactory intubating conditions are produced within 2.5 minutes; a single dose will last 10–20 minutes. The mean recovery index is 6.6 minutes. The drug is non-cumulative with repeated administration.

Effects
CVS Mivacurium has minimal cardiovascular effects; a slight (7%) transient decrease in blood pressure and slight (7%) increase in heart rate may occur after rapid intravenous injection. The drug has no significant vagal or ganglion blocking properties in the normal dosage range.
RS Neuromuscular blockade leads to apnoea; bronchospasm may occur secondary to histamine release.

Toxicity/Side Effects Transient cutaneous flushing is the most common side effect. Hypotension, tachycardia, bronchospasm and urticaria may all occur with an incidence of less than 1%. There have been rare reports of fatal anaphylactoid reactions with the administration of mivacurium. Cross-sensitivity may exist with vecuronium, rocuronium and pancuronium.

Kinetics

Distribution The V_D of the *trans-trans* isomer is 0.1 l/kg and that of the *cis-trans* isomer is 0.3 l/kg.

Metabolism The primary mechanism of metabolism of mivacurium is enzymatic hydrolysis by plasma cholinesterases to yield a quaternary alcohol and a quaternary monoester metabolite, which appear to be inactive. Some hydrolysis by liver esterases also occurs.

Excretion The metabolites are excreted in the bile and urine, together with some unchanged drug. The clearance of the *trans-trans* isomer is 53 ml/kg/minute and the elimination half-life is 2.3 minutes. The clearance of the *cis-trans* isomer is 92 ml/kg/minute and the elimination half-life is 2.1 minutes. Renal failure increases the clinical duration of action of mivacurium by a factor of 1.5 and hepatic failure increases it by a factor of 3.

Special Points The duration of action of mivacurium is prolonged by isoflurane and enflurane and to a lesser extent by halothane. The following drugs may enhance the neuromuscular effects of mivacurium: aminoglycoside antibiotics, propranolol, calcium channel blockers, diuretics, magnesium and lithium salts. The following drugs may reduce plasma cholinesterase activity and similarly enhance the activity of mivacurium: oral contraceptives, glucocorticoids and monoamine oxidase inhibitors.

Mivacurium does not act as a trigger agent for malignant hyperpyrexia in animal models.

The drug is physically incompatible with alkaline solutions (e.g. barbiturates).

Morphine

Uses Morphine is used:
1. for premedication
2. as an analgesic in the management of moderate to severe pain
3. in the treatment of left ventricular failure
4. to provide analgesia during terminal care and
5. in combination with kaolin in the symptomatic treatment of diarrhoea.

Chemical A phenanthrene derivative.

Presentation As 5/10/30/60/100/200 mg tablets, a syrup containing 2/10/20 mg/ml, as 15/30 mg suppositories and as a clear, colourless solution for injection containing 10/15/30 mg/ml of morphine sulphate, preservative-free morphine must be used for epidural/spinal use.

Main Actions Analgesia and respiratory depression.

Mode of Action Morphine is an agonist at mu- and kappa-opioid receptors. Opioids appear to exert their effects by increasing intracellular calcium concentration, which in turn increases potassium conductance and hyperpolarisation of excitable cell membranes. The decrease in membrane excitability that results may decrease both pre- and post-synaptic responses.

Routes of Administration/Doses The initial adult oral dose is 5–20 mg 4-hourly, increased as required. The dose by the rectal route is 15–30 mg 4-hourly. The corresponding intramuscular or subcutaneous dose is 0.1–0.2 mg/kg and the intravenous dose is 0.05–0.1 mg/kg 3–4 hourly. Morphine may also be administered intrathecally; an adult dose of 0.2–1 mg has been recommended. The drug has a peak analgesic effect 30–60 minutes after intramuscular injection and has a duration of effect of 3–4 hours.

Effects
CVS Morphine has minimal effects on the cardiovascular system; the predominant effect is that of orthostatic hypotension secondary to a decrease in the systemic vascular resistance, at least part of which is mediated by histamine release. The drug may also cause bradycardia when administered in high doses.
RS The principal effect of the drug is respiratory depression, with a decreased ventilatory response to hypoxia and hypercapnia. Morphine also has a potent antitussive action. Bronchoconstriction may occur with the use of high doses of the drug.

CNS Morphine is a potent analgesic agent, and may also cause drowsiness, relief of anxiety and euphoria. Miosis is produced by the drug as a result of stimulation of the Edinger-Westphal nucleus. Seizures and muscular rigidity may occur with the use of high doses of morphine.

AS Morphine decreases gastrointestinal motility and decreases gastric acid, biliary and pancreatic secretion; it also increases the common bile duct pressure by causing spasm of the sphincter of Oddi. The drug may also cause nausea, vomiting and constipation.

GU The drug increases the tone of the ureters, bladder detrusor muscle and sphincter and may precipitate urinary retention.

Metabolic/Other Mild diaphoresis and pruritus may result from histamine release. Morphine increases the secretion of ADH and may therefore lead to impaired water excretion and hyponatraemia. The drug causes a transient decrease in adrenal steroid secretion.

Toxicity/Side Effects Respiratory depression, nausea and vomiting, hallucinations and dependence may complicate the use of morphine. Pruritus may occur after epidural or spinal administration of the drug.

Kinetics

Absorption Morphine is well absorbed when administered orally, the bioavailability by this route is 15–50% due to an extensive first-pass metabolism.

Distribution The drug is 20–40% protein-bound in the plasma, predominantly to albumin; the V_D is 3.4–4.7 l/kg. Morphine equilibrates slowly between the plasma and CSF; there is no clear correlation between the degree of analgesia and the plasma concentration of the drug.

Metabolism Occurs in the liver to morphine-3-glucuronide, morphine-6-glucuronide and normorphine. In animal models morphine-6-glucuronide has analgesic effects and morphine-3-glucuronide has effects on arousal. Enterohepatic cycling of the metabolites probably does not occur.

Excretion Occurs predominantly in the urine as the glucuronide conjugates; 7–10% appears in the faeces as conjugated morphine. The clearance is 12–23 ml/min/kg and the elimination half-life is 1.7–4.5 hours. Cumulation of morphine-6-glucuronide occurs in the presence of renal failure; a reduction in the dose of the drug is necessary under these circumstances.

Special Points Morphine should be used with caution in the presence of hepatic failure, as the drug may precipitate encephalopathy. Similarly, the use of the drug in patients with hypopituitarism may precipitate coma. In common with

Morphine

other opioids, morphine decreases the apparent MAC of co-administered volatile agents. The actions of the drug are all reversed by naloxone, although the analgesia afforded by the epidural administration of morphine is well preserved after the administration of naloxone.

Morphine is not removed by haemodialysis or by peritoneal dialysis.

Nalbuphine

Uses Nalbuphine is used:
1. for premedication and
2. as an analgesic in the treatment of moderate to severe pain.

Chemical A semi-synthetic phenanthrene derivative.

Presentation As a clear, colourless solution for injection containing 10 mg/ml of nalbuphine hydrochloride.

Main Action Analgesia.

Mode of Action Nalbuphine is an agonist at kappa-opioid receptors and an antagonist at mu-opioid receptors; it thus produces analgesia (a kappa-effect) whilst antagonising both the respiratory depressant effects and the potential for dependency that are associated with the mu-receptor.

Routes of Administration/Doses The drug may be administered intravenously, intramuscularly or subcutaneously in an adult dose of 10–20 mg. Nalbuphine acts within 2–3 minutes when administered intravenously and within 15 minutes when administered intramuscularly. The duration of action is 3–6 hours.

Effects
CVS Nalbuphine has little significant effect on the heart rate, mean arterial pressure, systemic or pulmonary vascular resistance or cardiac output.
RS The drug has a respiratory depressant effect equal to that of morphine, but demonstrates a ceiling effect at a dose of 0.5 mg/kg. It will antagonise the respiratory depressant effects of co-administered pure mu-agonists, whilst adding to the analgesic effect of the latter.
CNS Nalbuphine has an analgesic potency equivalent to that of morphine. It has no euphoriant effects.
AS The drug causes less inhibition of gastrointestinal activity than other opioids.

Toxicity/Side Effects Sedation, dizziness, vertigo, dry mouth and headache may complicate the use of nalbuphine. The drug causes less nausea and vomiting, psychotomimetic effects and dependence than does morphine.

Kinetics

Absorption The bioavailability by the oral route is 12–17% due to a significant first-pass hepatic metabolism. The bioavailability is 80% by the intramuscular and subcutaneous routes.

Distribution Nalbuphine is 25–40% protein-bound in the plasma; the V_D is 162–498 l.

Metabolism Occurs predominantly in the liver to two inactive conjugates which are secreted into the bile.

Excretion The metabolites are predominantly excreted (with some unchanged nalbuphine) via the faeces. A small fraction is excreted unchanged in the urine. The clearance is 0.8–2.3 l/min and the elimination half-life is 110–160 minutes. Care should be exercised during the use of the drug in patients with renal or hepatic impairment.

Special Points Nalbuphine is ineffective in obtunding the cardiovascular responses to laryngoscopy and intubation. The drug will precipitate withdrawal symptoms in opiate addicts; its effects are reversed by naloxone.

Nalbuphine has been used in the management of postoperative shivering.

Naloxone

Uses Naloxone is used for:
1. the reversal of respiratory depression due to opioids
2. the diagnosis of suspected opioid overdose and has been used in the treatment of
3. clonidine overdose
4. obesity and
5. septic shock.

Chemical A substituted oxymorphone derivative.

Presentation As a clear solution for injection containing 0.02/0.4 mg/ml of naloxone hydrochloride.

Main Actions Reversal of mu-opioid receptor effects, i.e. sedation, hypotension, respiratory depression and the dysphoric effects of partial agonists. The drug will precipitate acute withdrawal symptoms in opiate addicts.

Mode of Action Naloxone is a competitive antagonist at mu-, delta-, kappa- and sigma-opioid receptors.

Routes of Administration/Doses For the reversal of opioid-induced respiratory depression, the drug should be administered intravenously in small incremental doses until the desired end point of reversal of respiratory depression without reversal of analgesia is reached; in adults, 0.1–0.2 mg will normally achieve this effect. In the treatment of known or suspected opioid overdose, 0.4–2.0 mg may be administered intravenously, intramuscularly or subcutaneously. The drug acts within 2 minutes when administered intravenously, and has a duration of effect (approximately 20 minutes) that may be shorter than the opioid whose effects it is desired to counteract. It may therefore be necessary to administer additional doses of naloxone intravenously or intramuscularly.

Effects
CVS The drug has no effect at normal doses; in doses >0.3 mg/kg the blood pressure may increase. Naloxone has been shown to reverse the hypotension associated with endotoxic and hypovolaemic shock in some animal studies.
CNS Naloxone causes slight drowsiness at very high doses. Some forms of stress-induced analgesia are obtunded by naloxone; the drug also decreases the tolerance to pain in subjects with high pain thresholds.
AS Naloxone reverses opioid-induced spasm of the sphincter of Oddi.

Toxicity/Side Effects There are two reports of serious ventricular dysrhythmias occurring in patients with irritable myocardia after the administration of naloxone.

Kinetics

Absorption   The drug is 91% absorbed when administered orally, but has a bioavailability by this route of 2%, due to an extensive first-pass metabolism.

Distribution   The drug is 46% protein-bound in adult plasma. The V_D is 2 l/kg.

Metabolism   The drug is metabolised in the liver, primarily by conjugation to glucuronide.

Excretion   The clearance is 25 ml/min/kg and the plasma half-life is 1.2 hours.

Special Points   Naloxone is effective in alleviating the pruritus, nausea and respiratory depression associated with the epidural or spinal administration of opioids.

Neostigmine

Uses   Neostigmine is used:
1. for the reversal of non-depolarising neuromuscular blockade and in the treatment of
2. myasthenia gravis
3. paralytic ileus and
4. urinary retention.

Chemical   A quaternary amine which is an ester of an alkyl carbamic acid.

Presentation   As 15 mg tables of neostigmine bromide and as a clear, colourless solution for injection containing 2.5 mg/ml of neostigmine metilsulfate. A fixed dose combination containing 0.5 mg of glycopyrronium and 2.5 mg of neostigmine metilsulfate per ml is also available.

Main Actions   Cholinergic.

Mode of Action   Neostigmine is a reversible, acid-transferring cholinesterase inhibitor which binds to the esteratic site of acetylcholinesterase and is hydrolysed by the latter, but at a much slower rate than is acetylcholine. The accumulation of acetylcholine at the neuromuscular junction allows the competitive antagonism of any non-depolarising relaxant that may be present.

Routes of Administration/Doses   The adult oral dose is 15–50 mg 2–4 hourly. The intravenous dose for the reversal of non-depolarising neuromuscular blockade is 0.05–0.07 mg/kg, administered slowly and in combination with an appropriate dose of an anticholinergic agent. The peak effect of the drug when administered intravenously occurs at 7–11 minutes; a single dose of neostigmine has a duration of action of 40–60 minutes.

Effects
CVS   The effects of neostigmine on the cardiovascular system are variable and depend upon the prevailing autonomic tone. The drug may cause bradycardia, leading to a fall in cardiac output; it decreases the effective refractory period of cardiac muscle and increases conduction time in conducting tissue. In high doses, neostigmine may cause hypotension secondary to a central effect.
RS   Neostigmine increases bronchial secretion and may cause bronchoconstriction.
CNS   In small doses, the drug has a direct action on skeletal muscle leading to muscular contraction. In high doses, neostigmine may block neuromuscular transmission by the combination of a direct effect and by allowing the accumulation of acetylcholine. Miosis and failure of accommodation may be precipitated by the administration of the drug.

AS The drug increases salivation, lower oesophageal and gastric tone, gastric acid output and lower gastrointestinal tract motility. Nausea and vomiting may occur.

GU Neostigmine increases ureteric peristalsis and may lead to involuntary micturition.

Metabolic/Other Sweating and lachrymation are increased.

Toxicity/Side Effects The side effects are manifestations of its pharmacological actions as described above. Cardiac arrest has been reported after the use of neostigmine.

Kinetics Data are incomplete.

Absorption Neostigmine is poorly absorbed when administered orally; the bioavailability by this route is 1–2%.

Distribution The drug is highly ionised and therefore does not cross the blood–brain barrier to any significant extent. Neostigmine is 6–10% protein-bound in the plasma, the V_D is 0.4–1 l/kg.

Metabolism Neostigmine is predominantly metabolised by plasma esterases to a quaternary alcohol; some hepatic metabolism with subsequent biliary excretion may also occur.

Excretion 50–67% of an administered dose is excreted in the urine. The clearance is 5.7–11.1 ml/min/kg and the elimination half-life is 15–80 minutes; the clearance is decreased and the elimination half-life is increased in the presence of renal impairment.

Special Points Neostigmine prolongs the duration of action of suxamethonium. There is some evidence that the use of neostigmine to reverse neuromuscular blockade is associated with an increased incidence of gastrointestinal anastamotic breakdown.

Nifedipine

Uses Nifedipine is used in the treatment of:
1. angina
2. mild to severe hypertension (including pregnancy-induced hypertension)
3. Raynaud's phenomenon and
4. coronary artery spasm occurring during coronary angiography or angioplasty.

Chemical A dihydropyridine derivative.

Presentation As 5/10 mg capsules and a slow-release preparation containing 10/20/30/60 mg per tablet. A fixed dose combination with atenolol is also available.

Main Actions Relaxation of arterial smooth muscle in both the coronary and peripheral circulations.

Mode of Action Nifedipine causes competitive blockade of cell membrane slow calcium channels leading to decreased influx of calcium ions into cells. This produces electromechanical decoupling, inhibition of contraction and relaxation of cardiac and smooth muscle fibres and leads to a negative inotropic effect and vasodilation. It may also act by increasing red cell deformability and preventing platelet clumping and thromboxane release.

Routes of Administration/Doses The adult oral dose of nifedipine is 10–20 mg 8-hourly (20–40 mg 12-hourly for the slow-release preparation), 100–200 µg may be infused via a coronary catheter over 2 minutes.

Effects
CVS The mean arterial pressure decreases by 20–33%; this effect is more pronounced in hypertensive patients. This is accompanied by a reflex increase in heart rate by up to 28%. The systemic and pulmonary vascular resistance, left ventricular end-diastolic and pulmonary artery pressure all decrease. Cardiac output is increased; nifedipine also causes a sustained relaxation of epicardial conductance vessels, leading to increased coronary blood flow in patients with ischaemic heart disease. Nifedipine is 3–10 times more effective in inhibiting contraction in coronary artery smooth muscle than in myocardial contractile cells. The drug may also protect the myocardium during reperfusion after cardiac bypass.
RS Nifedipine demonstrates no intrinsic bronchodilator effect in most studies. The drug appears to inhibit hypoxic pulmonary vasoconstriction.
CNS The drug causes a marginal increase in the cerebral blood flow due to vasodilation of large cerebral vessels.

AS Contractility throughout the gut and lower oesophageal pressure are decreased by nifedipine. The hepatic blood flow is increased.

GU Nifedipine has no marked effect on the renal blood flow or glomerular filtration rate. Uterine activity is decreased by the drug.

Metabolic/Other Plasma renin activity and catecholamines are increased; short-term use may decrease glucose tolerance. Platelet aggregation is impaired by the drug; thromboxane synthesis is inhibited and nifedipine may thus decrease thromboxane-induced coronary artery spasm.

Toxicity/Side Effects Occur in 20% of patients; head-ache, flushing and dizziness (secondary to vasodilation) are common; oedema of the legs, eye pain and gum hyperplasia have been reported.

Kinetics

Absorption Nifedipine is completely absorbed when administered orally; the bioavailability by this route is 45–68%.

Distribution The drug is 92–98% protein-bound in the plasma, the V_D is 0.62–1.12 l/kg.

Metabolism 95% of the dose is metabolised in the liver to three inactive metabolites.

Excretion 90% of the metabolites are excreted in the urine, the rest in the faeces. The clearance is 27–66 l/hour and the elimination half-life is 1.3–11 hours, dependent upon the route of administration.

Special Points Nifedipine is a safe and effective drug for the treatment of post-surgical hypertension; the reduction in mean arterial pressure is associated with an increase in cardiac index and systemic oxygen transport.

All volatile agents in current use decrease calcium ion release from the sarcoplasmic reticulum and decrease calcium ion flux into cardiac cells; the negatively inotropic effects of nifedipine are thus additive with those of the volatile agents. When used in combination with isoflurane, the negative inotropic effects of the drugs are additive and may result in a profound decrease in cardiac output.

Experiments in animals have demonstrated an increased risk of sinus arrest if volatile agents and calcium antagonists are used concurrently. If withdrawn acutely (especially in the post-operative period) after chronic oral use, severe rebound hypertension may result.

Calcium antagonists may also:
1. reduce the MAC of volatile agents by up to 20% and

Nifedipine

2. increase the efficacy of neuromuscular blocking agents.
    Administration of nifedipine immediately prior to induction appears to aggravate redistribution hypothermia.
    The drug is not removed by dialysis.

Nimodipine

Uses   Nimodipine is used:
1. in the prevention and treatment of cerebral vasospasm secondary to subarachnoid haemorrhage and may be of use in the management of
2. migraine
3. acute cerebrovasular accidents and
4. drug-resistant epilepsy.

Chemical   A dihydropyridine.

Presentation   As an intravenous infusion containing $200\,\mu g/ml$ of nimodipine and 30 mg tablets.

Main Action   Dilation of cerebral vessels leading to improved cerebral perfusion.

Mode of Action   Nimodipine is a calcium antagonist that binds to specific sites in the cell membranes of vascular smooth muscle and prevents calcium ion influx through 'slow' calcium ion channels, leading to vasodilation; the drug has a relatively specific action on cerebral arterioles.

Routes of Administration/Dose   The drug should be administered into a running crystalloid infusion via a central vein at the rate of 1 mg/hour for the first two hours and thereafter at the rate of 2 mg/hour for 5–14 days.

Effects
CVS   In normal subjects, doses of >2 mg/hour decrease the systolic and diastolic blood pressure. In the anaesthetised patient, an infusion of $1\,\mu g/kg/min$ decreases the systemic vascular resistance by 10–40% and increases cardiac output by 25–45%.
CNS   Nimodipine increases the cerebral blood flow by up to 18% with no demonstrable 'steal' effect in patients who have had a subarachnoid haemorrhage. The use of nimodipine in such patients leads to a significant reduction in mortality and morbidity.

Toxicity/Side Effects   Side effects occur infrequently, although flushing, headache, nausea, hypotension and reversible abnormalities of liver function tests may complicate the use of the drug.

Kinetics

Absorption   Nimodipine is rapidly and well absorbed when administered orally, but has a bioavailability by this route of only 3–28% due to a significant first-pass metabolism.

Distribution   The drug is 98% protein-bound in the plasma; the V_D is 0.94–2.3 l/kg.

Metabolism Nimodipine is initially demethylated and dehydrogenated to an inactive pyridine analogue which subsequently undergoes further degradation.

Excretion Half of the dose appears as metabolites in the urine, and a third in the faeces. The clearance is 420–520 l/hour and the elimination half-life is 0.9–7.2 hours (dependent upon the route of administration). The clearance is decreased by hepatic impairment; the effect of renal impairment is unclear.

Special Points Nimodipine has some effect in obtunding the cardiovascular responses to intubation and surgical stimulation; the peak blood pressures post-intubation and post-incision are consistently 10–15% lower in patients receiving the drug than those recorded in untreated patients.

The drug is adsorbed onto polyvinyl chloride tubing and is also light-sensitive; however, it remains stable in diffuse daylight for up to 10 hours.

Nitric oxide

Uses Nitric oxide (NO) is used as a selective pulmonary vasodilator in:
1. acute lung injury and
2. pulmonary hypertension and may be of use in the treatment of
3. bronchospasm and
4. chronic obstructive airways disease.

Chemical An inorganic gas.

Presentation In aluminium or stainless steel cylinders containing 100/1000/2000 p.p.m. nitric oxide in nitrogen; the cylinders are typically of 40 l capacity. Pure nitric oxide is toxic and corrosive. The gas is not licensed for use in the United Kingdom.

Main Action Vasodilation.

Mode of Action Nitric oxide is produced *in vivo* by NO synthase which uses the substrate L-arginine. Nitric oxide diffuses to the vascular smooth muscle layer and stimulates guanylate cyclase; the cGMP produced activates a phosphorylation cascade which leads to smooth muscle relaxation and vasodilation.

Route of Administration/Dose Nitric oxide is administered by inhalation in a dose of 5–80 p.p.m.; the drug is injected into the patient limb of the inspiratory circuit of a ventilator. The delivery system is designed to minimize the oxidation of nitric oxide to nitrogen dioxide. Monitoring of nitric oxide concentrations can be achieved by a chemiluminescent monitor or electrochemical detector.

Effects
CVS Nitric oxide is a potent vasodilator that mediates the hypotension and significant vascular leak characteristic of septic shock. Inhaled nitric oxide is a selective pulmonary vasodilator, since it is avidly bound to haemoglobin and thereby inactivated before reaching the systemic circulation. Nitric oxide released from vascular endothelium inhibits platelet aggregation and attenuates platelet and white cell adhesion. Inhaled nitrous oxide prolongs the bleeding time in volunteers.
RS Nitric oxide inhibits hypoxic pulmonary vasoconstriction and preferentially increases blood flow through well-ventilated areas of the lung, thereby improving ventilation:perfusion relationships.
CNS Nitric oxide increases cerebral blood flow and appears to have a physiological role as a neurotransmitter within the autonomic and central nervous systems.
AS Nitric oxide is a determinant of gastrointestinal motility and appears to modulate morphine-induced constipation.

GU Nitric oxide may play a role in the regulation of tenin production and sodium homeostasis in the kidney. It is the physiological mediator of penile erection.

Metabolic/Other Nitric oxide release from macrophages reacts with superoxide ion to form the free radical peroxynitrite, which is toxic to bacteria. Insulin release appears to be modulated by nitric oxide.

Toxicity/Side Effects Exposure to 500–2000 p.p.m of nitric oxide results in methaemoglobinaemia and pulmonary oedema. Contamination by nitrogen dioxide can similarly lead to pneumonitis and pulmonary oedema.

Kinetics

Absorption Nitric oxide is highly lipid soluble and diffuses freely across cell membranes.

Metabolism The gas is rapidly converted to nitrates and nitrites in the presence of oxygen. Inhaled nitric oxide readily reacts with oxidised haemoglobin to yield methaemoglobin; nitric oxide has a half-life <5 seconds.

Special Points Prolonged inhalation (up to 27 days) of the gas appears safe and is not associated with tachyphylaxis.

Abrupt cessation of nitric oxide can cause a profound decrease in P_aO_2 and increase in pulmonary artery pressure, possibly via down-regulation of endogenous NO production or guanylate cyclase activity.

Mortality does not appear to be affected by the administration of NO in ARDS.

Nitrous oxide

Uses   Nitrous oxide is used:
1. as an adjuvant to general anaesthesia
2. as an analgesic during labour and other painful procedures and
3. for cryotherapy.

Chemical   An inorganic gas.

Presentation   As a liquid in cylinders at a pressure of 44 bar at 15 °C; the cylinders are blue and are available in five sizes (C–G, containing 450–9000 l respectively). Nitrous oxide is a colourless gas with a sweet smell; it is non-flammable but does support combustion. The specific gravity of the gas is 1.53, the boiling point −88°C, the critical temperature 36.5°C and the critical pressure 71.7 atmospheres. The MAC of nitrous oxide is 105, the oil/water solubility coefficient 3.2 and the blood/gas solubility coefficient is 0.47.

Entonox is the trade name given to a 50/50 mixture of oxygen and nitrous oxide. It is available in cylinders which are blue with white shoulders and are of two sizes (G and J, containing 3200 and 6400 l respectively). At normal temperatures, both of the components of Entonox are present in pressurised cylinders in the gaseous phase (due to the Poynting effect); liquefaction of nitrous oxide and separation of the two components may occur at temperatures of −7°C.

Main Actions   Analgesia and depression of the central nervous system.

Mode of Action   The mode of action of nitrous oxide is unknown; it may act by modulation of enkephalins and endorphins within the central nervous system.

Route of Administration/Dose   Nitrous oxide is administered by inhalation; a concentration of 70% in oxygen is conventionally used as a adjunct to general anaesthesia. Entonox is used to provide analgesia for a range of painful procedures.

Effects
CVS   Nitrous oxide decreases myocardial contractility *in vitro*; *in vivo*, the mean arterial pressure is usually well maintained by a reflex increase in peripheral vascular resistance. A deterioration in left ventricular function occurs when nitrous oxide is added to a high-dose opioid oxygen anaesthetic sequence, volatile agents or a propofol infusion.
RS   The gas causes a slight depression of respiration, with an attendant decrease in tidal volume and increase in respiratory rate. Nitrous oxide is non-irritant and does not cause bronchospasm.

CNS   Nitrous oxide is a central nervous system depressant and when administered in a concentration of 80% will cause loss of consciousness in most subjects. The gas is a powerful analgesic in concentrations of >20%. The administration of nitrous oxide increases intracranial pressure.

GU   Nitrous oxide has no effect on uterine tone.

Toxicity/Side Effects   15% of patients receiving nitrous oxide will experience nausea and vomiting. The gas is 35 times more soluble than nitrogen in the blood; nitrous oxide will therefore cause an increase in the size of air-filled spaces (e.g. pneumothorax, intestines, air cysts and the middle ear) in the body. A further manifestation of this physical property of the gas is the Fink effect (diffusion hypoxia): when nitrous oxide is discontinued, the ingress of the gas into the alveoli lowers the alveolar oxygen concentration. The prolonged use of high concentrations of nitrous oxide (>6 hours) leads to inactivation of the cobalamin component of methionine synthetase and to a reduction in thymidine and DNA synthesis. The resultant clinical syndrome is akin to pernicious anaemia; megaloblastic anaemia and pancytopenia. Protracted use of the gas may also lead to the development of a peripheral neuropathy. Nitrous oxide is teratogenic in animals when administered during early pregnancy.

Kinetics

Absorption   Nitrous oxide diffuses freely across the normal alveolar epithelium. The rate of uptake of the gas is increased by a decreased cardiac output, an increased concentration and by increased alveolar ventilation. Due to its relative insolubility, the alveolar concentration of nitrous oxide approaches the inspired concentration fairly rapidly; 90% equilibration occurring within 15 minutes and 100% equilibration within 5 hours.

Metabolism   Little, if any, metabolism occurs in man.

Excretion   Nitrous oxide is excreted unchanged through the lungs and skin.

Special Points   Nitrous oxide exhibits both the concentration and second gas effects. The concentration effect implies that the greater inspired anaesthetic concentration, the more rapid will be the rise in alveolar concentration. The second gas effect refers to the ability of one gas administered in a high concentration (e.g. nitrous oxide) to accelerate the uptake of another gas (e.g. halothane) that is administered simultaneously, the rapid absorption of the nitrous oxide increasing the alveolar concentration of the halothane.

70% nitrous-oxide in oxygen decreases the MAC of halothane to 0.29, that of enflurane to 0.6 and of isoflurane to 0.5. The use of nitrous oxide appears to be safe in patients susceptible to malignant hyperthermia.

Norepinephrine

Uses   Norepinephrine is used in the treatment of refractory hypotension.

Chemical   A catecholamine.

Presentation   As a clear, colourless solution containing 2 mg/ml of norepinephrine bitartrate for dilution prior to infusion.

Main Action   Increased systemic vascular resistance.

Mode of Action   Norepinephrine is a directly and indirectly acting sympathomimetic amine that exerts its action predominantly at alpha-adrenergic receptors, with a minor action at beta-receptors.

Route of Administration/Dose   Norepinephrine is administered through a central vein as an infusion in dextrose or saline in a concentration of 4 μg/ml at a rate titrated according to the response desired. The drug has a duration of action of 30–40 minutes; tachyphylaxis occurs with prolonged administration.

Effects
CVS   Norepinephrine increases the peripheral vascular resistance, leading to an increase in the systolic and diastolic blood pressure; the cardiac output remains unchanged or decreases slightly. Reflex vagal stimulation leads to a compensatory bradycardia. The drug produces coronary vasodilation leading to a marked increase in coronary blood flow. The circulating blood volume is reduced by norepinephrine, due to loss of protein-free fluid to the extracellular fluid. Norepinephrine may also cause nodal rhythm, atrio-ventricular dissociation and ventricular dysrhythmias.
RS   The drug causes a slight increase in the minute volume accompanied by a degree of bronchodilatation.
CNS   The cerebral blood flow and oxygen consumption are decreased by the administration of norepinephrine; mydriasis also occurs.
AS   The hepatic and splanchnic blood flow are decreased by the drug.
GU   Norepinephrine decreases the renal blood flow; the glomerular filtration rate is usually well maintained. The tone of the bladder neck is increased. Norepinephrine increases the contactility of the pregnant uterus; this may lead to fetal bradycardia and asphyxia.
Metabolic/Other   Norepinephrine may decrease insulin secretion, leading to hyperglycaemia; the concentration of free fatty acids and the plasma renin activity may increase.

Toxicity/Side Effects Anxiety, headache, photophobia, pallor, sweating, gangrene and chest pain may occur with the use of the drug. Extravasation of norepinephrine may lead to sloughing and tissue necrosis.

Kinetics

Absorption Norepinephrine undergoes significant first-pass metabolism and is inactive when administered orally.

Distribution The V_D is 0.09–0.4 l/kg.

Metabolism Exogenous norepinephrine is metabolised by two pathways; by oxidative deamination to the aldehyde by mitochondrial monoamine oxidase (in liver, brain and kidney) and by methylation by cytoplasmic catechol-O-methyl-transferase to normetanephrine. The predominant metabolite appearing in the urine is 3-methoxy, 4-hydroxymandelic acid (VMA).

Excretion 5% of an administered dose of norepinephrine is excreted unchanged; the clearance is 27.9–100 ml/min/kg and the half-life is 0.57–2.4 minutes.

Special Points The use of norepinephrine during halothane anaesthesia may lead to the appearance of serious cardiac dysrhythmias; if co-administered with MAOIs or tri-cyclic anti-depressants, serious hypertensive episodes may be precipitated.

The drug is pharmaceutically incompatible with barbiturates and sodium bicarbonate.

Omeprazole

Uses Omeprazole is used in the treatment of:
1. peptic ulcer disease
2. peptic oesophagitis and
3. the Zollinger-Ellison syndrome.

Chemical A substituted benzimidazole derivative.

Presentation As capsules containing 10/20/40 mg of omeprazole and in 40 mg vials as a powder of the sodium salt of omeprazole.

Main Actions Inhibition of basal and stimulated gastric acid secretion.

Mode of Action Omeprazole acts via a derivative which binds irreversibly to parietal cell H^+-K^+-ATPase and non-competitively inhibits it. The activity of the parietal cell 'proton pump', which represents the final common pathway of H^+ secretion, is thus inhibited.

Route of Administration/Doses The adult oral dose for the treatment of peptic ulcer disease is 20–40 mg daily for a period of 4–8 weeks; the corresponding dose for the treatment of the Zollinger-Ellison syndrome is 20–120 mg daily. The intravenous dose is administered over 5 minutes.

Effects
AS Omeprazole significantly reduces the volume of gastric juice but has no effect on the rate of gastric emptying. A single 20 mg dose will effectively control acid secretion for 24 hours. In animals, orally administered omeprazole appears to confer protection against stress-induced gastric ulceration.
Metabolic/Other The drug has no demonstrable effect on endocrine function.

Toxicity/Side Effects Omeprazole is usually well tolerated; rashes, nausea, headache, gastrointestinal disturbances, liver dysfunction and arrhythmia may occur.

Kinetics

Absorption Oral omeprazole is rapidly absorbed and has a bioavailability of 40–97%, dependent upon the formulation and dose. The drug may increase its own bioavailability, since degradation occurs under acidic conditions.

Distribution The drug is 95–96% protein-bound in the plasma, predominantly to albumin and alpha-1-acid glycoprotein. The V_D is 0.3–0.4 l/kg.

Metabolism Omperazole is rapidly and completely metabolised by oxidation to a sulphone, reduction to a sulphide and by hydroxylation.

Excretion 80% of an oral dose is excreted in the urine, the remainder in the faeces. The clearance is 533–666 ml/min and the elimination half-life is 0.5–1.5 hours.

Special Points Omeprazole is 2–10 times as potent as cimetidine; furthermore, it heals ulcers significantly more rapidly than conventional H_2-antagonist regimes and may be effective in patients resistant to conventional therapy.

The pharmacokinetics of the drug are unaltered by renal impairment and it is not removed by haemodialysis; no dose reduction is required in patients with renal or hepatic impairment. Omeprazole decreases the clearance of co-administered diazepam, phenytoin and warfarin.

The role of omeprazole in the prevention of stress ulceration in critically ill patients remains to be evaluated. The value of omeprazole in anaesthetic premedication is questionable.

Ondansetron

Uses   Ondansetron is used:
1. in the management of nausea and vomiting induced by chemotherapy and radiotherapy and
2. in the prevention and treatment of post-operative nausea and vomiting.

Chemical   A synthetic carbazole.

Presentation   As a clear, colourless aqueous solution in 2/4 ml ampoules containing 2 mg/ml ondansetron hydrochloride dihydrate and as 4/8 mg tablets.

Main Action   Antiemetic.

Mode of Action   Ondansetron is a highly selective antagonist at $5-HT_3$ receptors and acts both centrally and peripherally. Emetogenic stimuli appear to cause release of 5-HT in the small intestine and initiate a vomiting reflex by activating vagal afferents via $5-HT_3$ receptors; ondansetron blocks the initiation of this reflex. Activation of vagal afferents may also result in release of 5-HT in the area postrema, promoting emesis via a central mechanism.

Routes of Administration/Doses   For the management of post-operative nausea and vomiting, the adult dose is 8 mg 8-hourly orally or a single intramuscular or intravenous dose of 4 mg.

Effects
CVS   Ondansetron has no demonstrable effects on the cardiovascular system.
RS   The drug has no effect on the ventilatory response to CO_2.
CNS   Ondansetron has no sedative effects and does not impair performance in psychomotor tests.
AS   The drug has no effect on gastric motility, but does increase large bowel transit time.
Mecabolic/Other   Ondansetron has no effect on serum prolactin concentration or haemostatic function.

Toxicity/Side Effects   Constipation, headache and flushing may occur. Anaphylaxis has also been reported.

Kinetics

Absorption   Ondansetron is rapidly absorbed after oral administration and has a bioavailability of 60%.

Distribution   The drug is 76% protein-bound in the plasma; the V_D is 2 l/kg.

Metabolism   Ondansetron is extensively metabolised by hydroxylation or N-demethylation of the indole nucleus, followed by conjugation with glucuronic acid or sulphate.

Excretion   Less than 5% is excreted unchanged in the urine. The clearance is 6.3 ml/min/kg and the elimination half-life is 3 hours.

Special Points   No alteration of dose is needed in patients with renal impairment; hepatic impairment significantly prolongs the serum half-life of ondansetron and the dose should be limited to 8 mg/day.

Ondansetron may reduce the incidence of post-anaesthetic shivering.

Oxygen

Uses Oxygen is used:
1. in the management of all forms of hypoxia (other than histotoxic)
2. as an adjunct in the management of shock and in the treatment of
3. carbon monoxide poisoning
4. pneumatosis coli
5. decompression sickness and
6. anaerobic infections.

Chemical A gaseous inorganic element.

Presentation As a compressed gas in cylinders at a pressure of 137 bar at 15°C; the cylinders are black with white shoulders and are available in six sizes (C–J, containing 170–88001 respectively). Oxygen is also available commercially in liquid form, one volume of liquid oxygen yielding 840 volumes of gaseous oxygen.

Oxygen is a colourless, odourless, tasteless gas which supports combustion and is explosive in the presence of grease. The specific gravity of the gas is 1.105, the critical temperature −118.4°C and the critical pressure 50.8 atmospheres.

Main Action Oxygen's essential role is in the process of oxidative phosphorylation.

Mode of Action Elemental oxygen is combined with hydrogen ions via mitochondrial cytochrome oxidase; the energy released is used for the synthesis of ATP.

Route of Administration Oxygen is administered by inhalation; many devices are used for its administration and inspired concentrations of up to 100% may be achieved.

Effects
CVS The administration of 100% oxygen causes a slight decrease in the heart rate (due to an effect on chemoreceptors), a slight increase in diastolic blood pressure and a decrease of 8–20% in cardiac output, due to myocardial depression. The coronary blood flow decreases secondary to coronary arterial vasoconstriction. In contrast, the pulmonary vascular resistance and the mean pulmonary artery pressure decrease.
RS Mild respiratory depression (due to a decrease in sensitivity of the respiratory centre to carbon dioxide) results from the administration of 100% oxygen. Nitrogen is eliminated from the lungs within 2 minutes (leading to atelectasis subsequent to the loss of the 'splinting' effect of nitrogen), from the blood within 5 minutes and from the body within 2 hours. The binding of oxygen with haemoglobin tends to displace carbon dioxide from the blood (the Haldane effect).

CNS The administration of 100% oxygen causes cerebrovascular constriction (due to an increased sensitivity to adrenergic agonists), resulting in a decrease in cerebral blood flow.

Metabolic/Other The administration of 100% oxygen has no effect on glucose utilisation or the respiratory quotient.

Toxicity/Side Effects The following toxic effects are associated with the use of high concentrations of oxygen:

1. carbon dioxide retention in patients with respiratory failure who are predominantly dependent upon a hypoxic drive to respiration
2. retrolental fibroplasia
3. acute oxygen toxicity (the Paul-Bert effect) may occur if hyperbaric 100% oxygen is used; the symptoms are altered mood, vertigo, loss of consciousness and convulsions
4. chronic oxygen toxicity may occur when concentrations >60% are used for prolonged periods at atmospheric pressure; the symptoms of this are tracheal irritation, sore throat, substernal pain and the signs are pulmonary congestion, atelectasis and a decreased vital capacity
5. prolonged administration of 100% oxygen may interfere with red cell formation.

Kinetics

Absorption The gas is freely permeable through normal alveolar tissue.

Distribution Oxygen is transported in the blood predominantly combined to haemoglobin; in addition each 100 ml of plasma contains 0.3 ml of dissolved oxygen at normal atmospheric pressure and an FiO_2 of 0.21.

Metabolism Occurs within mitochondria to produce carbon dioxide and water.

Excretion As exhaled carbon dioxide and metabolic water.

Oxytocin

Uses Oxytocin is used:
1. for the induction and acceleration of labour
2. to promote lactation and in the management of
3. missed and incomplete abortion and
4. post-partum haemorrhage.

Chemical A naturally occurring polypeptide from the posterior lobe of the pituitary gland.

Presentation As a clear solution for injection containing 5/10 Units/ml of synthetic oxytocin (which is free from vasopressin and extraneous animal protein) and in a fixed dose combination for injection containing 5 Units/ml of oxytocin and 500 μg of ergometrine maleate (which has a more sustained effect on the uterus than does oxytocin).

Main Action Stimulation of uterine contraction.

Mode of Action Oxytocin is thought to act by binding to specific receptors on smooch muscle cells and increasing the permeability of the myometrial cell membrane to potassium ions, thereby decreasing the membrane potential and increasing the excitability of uterine smooth muscle.

Routes of Administration/Doses Oxytocin is administered by intravenous infusion at a rate of 1.5–12 mUnits/min, titrated against the frequency and duration of uterine contractions. The intramuscular dose of the oxytocin–ergometrine preparation is 1 ml.

Effects
CVS Bolus intravenous administration of oxytocin causes a decrease in the blood pressure that occurs within 30 seconds and lasts up to 10 minutes – this response is exaggerated in the anaesthetised subject. A reflex tachycardia and an increase in cardiac output by up to 1.5 l/min occur. ECG changes such as prolongation of the Q-T interval and T-wave flattening may reflect poor coronary artery filling.
AS Oxytocin has no effect on lower oesophageal sphincter pressure during pregnancy.
GU Infusions of oxytocin increase the renal blood flow in animal models.
Metabolic/Other Oxytocin has an antidiuretic effect (exerted by a direct action on the renal tubules) which may, when it is administered in high doses with large volumes of electrolyte-free fluid, lead to water intoxication. Oxytocin also causes milk ejection by causing contraction of modified smooth muscle within the mammary gland, forcing milk from alveolar channels into large sinuses.

Toxicity/Side Effects Oxytocin may cause uterine spasm and rupture, leading to fetal asphyxia when infused too rapidly. Anaphylactoid reactions to the drug have also been reported. Water intoxication has been described above.

Kinetics   Data are incomplete.

Absorption   Oxytocin is active when administered by any parenteral route, but is inactivated by chymotrypsin when administered orally.

Metabolism   Oxytocin is rapidly removed from the plasma by hydrolysis in the liver and kidney (by the action of oxytocinase).

Excretion   The elimination half-life is 1–7 minutes.

Special Points   Oxytocin should not be infused through the same intravenous line as blood and plasma as rapid inactivation of the polypeptide by plasma oxytocinase occurs. Infusions of oxytocin may alter the action of co-administered suxamethonium, leading to a decrease in the fasciculations caused by the latter and an increased dose requirement for suxamethonium.

Pancuronium

Uses Pancuronium is used to facilitate intubation and controlled ventilation.

Chemical A bis-quaternary aminosteroid.

Presentation As a clear solution for injection containing 2 mg/ml of pancuronium bromide.

Main Action Competitive neuromuscular blockade.

Mode of Action Pancuronium acts by competitive antagonism of acetylcholine at nicotinic (N2) receptors at the post-synaptic membrane of the neuromuscular junction; it also has some pre-junctional action.

Route of Administration/Dose Pancuronium is administered intravenously; the normal intubating dose is 0.05–0.1 mg/kg with subsequent doses of one-third this amount. Satisfactory intubating conditions are produced within 90–150 seconds according to the dose administered; a single dose lasts 45–60 minutes. The recovery index of the drug is 16–22 minutes.

Effects
CVS Pancuronium causes an increase in the heart rate, blood pressure and cardiac output secondary to a vagolytic action. The systemic vascular resistance remains unchanged after the administration of the drug.
RS Neuromuscular blockade results in apnoea. Pancuronium has a very low potential for histamine release; bronchospasm is extremely uncommon.
Metabolic/Other Pancuronium may decrease the partial thromboplastin time and prothrombin time.

Toxicity/Side Effects There have been rare reports of fatal anaphylactoid reactions with the administration of pancuronium. Cross-sensitivity may exist with vecuronium and rocuronium.

Kinetics

Distribution Pancuronium is 15–30% protein-bound in the plasma, predominantly to albumin and gamma globulin; the V_D is 0.134–0.162 l/kg. The drug does not cross the placental or blood–brain barrier.

Metabolism 30–45% of an administered dose undergoes hepatic metabolism by deacetylation to 3-hydroxy-, 17-hydroxy- and 3,17-dihydroxy-derivatives with subsequent biliary excretion. The 3-hydroxy-derivative has some neuromuscular-blocking activity.

Excretion   50% of the dose is excreted in the urine (80% of this as the unchanged drug), with 5–10% appearing in the bile. The clearance is 1.46–2.22 ml/min/kg and the elimination half-life is 69–129 minutes. The dose should be reduced in the presence of renal or hepatic impairment.

Special Points   The duration of action of pancuronium, in common with other non-depolarising relaxants, is prolonged by hypokalaemia, hypocalcaemia, hypermagnesaemia, hypoproteinaemia, dehydration, acidosis and hypercapnia. Conversely, pancuronium appears to decrease the MAC of halothane; it also tends to counteract the depressant effect of halothane on the blood pressure.

The following drugs, when co-administered with non-depolarising relaxants, increase the effect of the latter: volatile and induction agents, fentanyl, suxamethonium, diuretics, calcium antagonists, alpha- and beta-adenergic antagonists, protamine, metronidazole and the aminoglycoside antibiotics.

The use of pancuronium appears to be safe in patients susceptible to malignant hyperpyrexia.

Papaveretum

Uses   Papaveretum is used:
1. for premedication
2. as an analgesic in the management of moderate to severe pain and
3. to provide analgesia during terminal care.

Chemical   Papaveretum is a standardised mixture of the anhydrous hydrochlorides of the alkaloids of opium. It contains 253 parts of morphine hydrochloride, 23 parts of papaverine and 20 parts of codeine.

Presentation   As a clear, colourless solution for injection containing 7.7/15.4 mg/ml of papaveretum. A fixed-dose combination with scopolamine is also available.

Main Actions   Analgesia and respiratory depression.

Mode of Action   The activity of papaveretum is essentially that of morphine, which is an agonist at mu- and kappa-opioid receptors. Opioids appear to exert their effects by increasing intracellular calcium concentration, which in turn increases potassium conductance and hyperpolarisation of excitable cell membranes. The decrease in membrane excitability that results may decrease both pre- and post-synaptic responses.

Routes of Administration/Doses   The adult intramuscular or intravenous dose is 7.7/15.4 mg/kg 3–4 hourly. Papaveretum is not recommended for intrathecal or epidural administration, due to the presence of hydroxy-benzoate preservatives.

Effects
CVS   Papaveretum has minimal effects on the cardiovascular system; the predominant effect is that of orthostatic hypotension secondary to a decrease in the systemic vascular resistance, at least part of which is mediated by histamine release. The drug may also cause bradycardia when administered in high doses.
RS   The principal effect of the drug is respiratory depression, with a decreased ventilatory response to hypoxia and hypercapnia. Papaveretum also has a potent antitussive action. Bronchoconstriction may occur with the use of high doses of the drug.
CNS   Papaveretum is a potent analgesic agent, and may also cause sedation (to a greater degree than does morphine), relief of anxiety and euphoria. Miosis is produced by the drug as a result of stimulation of the Edinger-Westphal nucleus. Seizures and muscular rigidity may occur with the use of high doses of papaveretum.
AS   Papaveretum decreases gastrointestinal motility and decreases gastric acid, biliary and pancreatic secretion; it also

increases the common bile duct pressure by causing spasm of the sphincter of Oddi. The drug may also cause nausea and vomiting (although to a lesser extent than does morphine) and constipation.

GU   The drug increases the tone of the ureters, bladder detrusor muscle and sphincter and may precipitate urinary retention. **Metabolic/Other**   Mild diaphoresis and pruritus may result from histamine release. Papaveretum increases the secretion of ADH and may therefore lead to impaired water excretion and hyponatraemia. The drug causes a transient decrease in adrenal steroid secretion.

Toxicity/Side Effects   Respiratory depression, nausea and vomiting, hallucinations and dependence may complicate the use of papaveretum.

Kinetics   The kinetics of papaveretum are essentially those of morphine (q.v.).

Special Points   Papaveretum should be used with caution in the presence of hepatic failure, as the drug may precipitate encephalopathy. Similarly, the use of the drug in patients with hypopituitarism may precipitate coma. In common with other opioids, papaveretum decreases the apparent MAC of co-administered volatile agents. The actions of the drug are all reversed by naloxone.

Paracetamol

Uses Paracetamol is used:
1. as an analgesic for the relief of pain of mild to moderate severity and
2. as an antipyretic agent.

Chemical An acetanilide derivative.

Presentation As tablets and suppositories containing 120/500 mg of paracetamol and a syrup containing 24/50 mg/ml. A number of fixed dose combinations with dextropropoxyphene, codeine, pentazocine or metaclopramide are also available.

Main Actions Analgesic and antipyretic.

Mode of Action The mode of action of paracetamol is poorly understood. It is apparently a potent inhibitor of prostaglandin synthesis within the central nervous system which accounts for its antipyretic effect – specifically, it inhibits the synthesis of the E series of prostaglandins that are normally produced in the anterior hypothalamus in response to pyrogens. It acts peripherally by blocking impulse generation within the bradykinin-sensitive chemoreceptors responsible for the generation of afferent nociceptive impulses.

Routes of Administration/Doses The adult oral and rectal dose is 500 mg–1 g 4–6 hourly. Analgesic in children may require 90 mg/kg/day in divided doses (30 mg/kg per dose).

Effects
CNS The maximum analgesic effect of paracetamol appears to be greater than that of any other non-opioid analgesic.
AS Paracetamol is occasionally used as a model for drug absorption as its rate of absorption is proportional to the gastric emptying rate. Drugs which alter gastric emptying alter the rate of paracetamol absorption. The drug has no effect on the liver unless taken in overdose and does not cause gastric ulceration.
Metabolic/Other The drug potentiates the effect of antidiuretic hormone. It has no effect on normal haemostatic mechanisms.

Toxicity/Side Effects Gastrointestinal disturbances, skin reactions and idiosyncratic haemopoietic disorders (thrombocytopenia) may occur with therapeutic doses. Approximately 5% of patients who are allergic to aspirin show cross-sensitivity to paracetamol.

Kinetics

Absorption The drug is rapidly absorbed from the upper gastrointestinal tract; the bioavailability when administered by the oral route is 70–90% due to first-pass metabolism. Absorption is variable when administered rectally and the bioavailability by this route is 68–88% of that observed after oral administration.

Distribution At therapeutic levels, paracetamol is 0–5% protein-bound in the plasma; the V_D is 1 l/kg. Being a non-ionised, lipid soluble substance, paracetamol penetrates tissues and the blood–brain barrier well.

Metabolism Occurs predominantly in the liver, 80% being metabolised to glucuronide and sulphate and 10% by cytochrome P-450 to a highly reactive intermediate metabolite which is in turn inactivated by conjugation with glutathione.

Excretion 2–5% is excreted unchanged in the urine; the glucuronide and sulphate metabolites are actively secreted in the renal tubules at low concentrations and actively reabsorbed at high concentrations. The clearance is 5 ml/min/kg and the elimination half-life is 1.9 hours.

Special Points Paracetamol should be used with caution in patients with renal or hepatic impairment.

Hepatic damage occurs readily with doses exceeding 15 g of the drug; with toxic doses the supply of glutathione becomes depleted and the highly reactive intermediate metabolite of paracetamol combines with hepatic cell membranes, leading eventually to centrilobular necrosis. N-acetylcysteine and methionine act as alternative supplies of glutathione and can protect against paracetamol-induced liver damage if administered within 10–12 hours of ingestion of paracetamol. Liver function tests are a poor prognostic indicator under these circumstances; bilirubin levels >4 mg/100 ml and an INR of >2.2 are associated with a poor outcome.

Penicillin

Uses   Penicillin is used in the treatment of infections of:
1. the respiratory tract
2. ear, nose and throat
3. skin, bone, soft tissues and wounds and in the treatment of
4. gonorrhoea
5. meningitis and
6. subacute bacterial endocarditis.

Chemical   The prototype penicillin.

Presentation   The preparation for oral use is phenoxymethylpenicillin (penicillin V), which is presented as 125/250 mg tablets and in an elixir as the potassium salt. The parenteral preparation is benzylpenicillin (penicillin G), which is a white crystalline powder presented in vials containing 0.3/0.6/3/6 g of sodium benzylpenicillin.

Main Actions   Penicillin is a bactericidal antibiotic with a narrow spectrum of activity which includes *Streptococcus, Neisseria, Haemophilus, Corynebacterium, Bacillus, Clostridium, Listeria* and *Treponema* sp., some sensitive staphylococcal strains and oral anaerobes. Penicillin is destroyed by beta-lactamases produced by some strains of *Pseudomonas*, Enterobacteriaceae and *Bacteroides*.

Mode of Action   Penicillin binds specifically to penicillin-binding proteins (transpeptidases and carboxypeptidases) in the bacterial cell wall and prevents peptidoglycan cross-linking, thereby decreasing the mechanical stability of the bacterial cell wall.

Routes of Administration/Doses   The adult oral dose is 125–250 mg 4–6 hourly; the corresponding intravenous and intramuscular dose is 0.6–4.8 g/day in 2–4 divided doses. 1 megaUnit is 600 mg. Penicillin may also be administered intrathecally.

Effects
Metabolic/Other   High doses of benzylpenicillin may produce hypernatraemia and hypokalaemia.

Toxicity/Side Effects   Gastrointestinal disturbances, allergic phenomena (including anaphylaxis), rashes and haemolytic anaemia may occur with the use of the drug. High parenteral doses of penicillin may cause neuropathy and nephropathy.

Kinetics

Absorption   15–30% of an oral dose of penicillin G (the drug is unstable under acid conditions) and 60% of an oral dose of penicillin V is absorbed. The pharmacokinetics after absorption are similar for both preparations.

Distribution Penicillin is 59–67% protein-bound in the plasma, predominantly to albumin; the V_D is 0.32–0.81 l/kg.

Metabolism Penicillin is metabolised to penicilloic acid which is inactive with subsequent transformation to penamaldic and penicillenic acid.

Excretion 60–90% of a dose is excreted in the urine by active tubular secretion; up to 25% is excreted unchanged. The elimination half-life is 0.7 hours.

Special Points Penicillin is removed by haemodialysis.

Pentazocine

Uses Pentazocine is used for the relief of moderate to severe pain.

Chemical A benzmorphan derivative.

Presentation As tablets containing 25/50 mg of pentazocine hydrochloride, as 50 mg suppositories, and a clear solution for injection containing 30 mg/ml of pentazocine lactate.

Main Action Analgesia.

Mode of Action Pentazocine appears to exert its analgesic effects by an agonistic effect at kappa-opioid receptors; it has weak antagonistic activity at mu-opioid receptors.

Routes of Administration/Doses The adult oral dose is 50–100 mg 3–4 hourly; the corresponding parenteral dose is 30–60 mg 3–4 hourly. The drug is irritant when injected intramuscularly or subcutaneously. Pentazocine acts within 2–3 minutes when administered intravenously and within 20 minutes when administered intramuscularly; the duration of action is 3–4 hours.

Effects
CVS High doses of the drug may lead to a slight increase in the heart rate and blood pressure; this may lead to an increase in cardiac work.

RS Pentazocine causes an equal degree of respiratory depression as an equipotent dose of morphine; however, a 'ceiling effect' limits the degree of respiratory depression produced with doses in excess of 60 mg.

CNS The drug is approximately one-third as potent an analgesic as morphine; it cause sedation and does not exhibit any euphoriant properties.

AS Pentazocine appears to cause less nausea and vomiting and a less marked rise in biliary tract pressure than an equipotent dose of morphine. The drug decreases both gastric and small intestinal motility.

GU Pentazocine decreases the renal plasma flow but has no effect on glomerular filtration rate. The drug increases uterine activity.

Metabolic/Other The drug causes an increase in the plasma catecholamine concentration.

Toxicity/Side Effects Respiratory depression, dizziness, nausea, sweating, dysphoria and hallucinations may complicate the use of the drug. Tolerance and dependence may occur with prolonged use.

Kinetics

Absorption   The drug is well absorbed when administered orally; the bioavailability is 20% due to a significant hepatic first-pass metabolism.

Distribution   Pentazocine is 60–70% protein-bound in the plasma; the V_D is 4.9 l/kg.

Metabolism   Occurs in the liver by oxidation and glucuronidation.

Excretion   60% of the dose is excreted in the urine within 24 hours, 2–12% unchanged. The clearance is 1320 ml/min and the elimination half-life is 2 hours.

Special Points   Pentazocine, being a weak antagonist at mu-opioid receptors, can precipitate withdrawal symptoms in opiate addicts. The respiratory depressant effects of the drug are reversed by naloxone.

Pentazocine is pharmaceutically incompatible with thiopentone, methohexitone and diazepam.

The drug is removed by haemodialysis.

Pethidine

Uses   Pethidine is used:
1. for premedication
2. as an analgesic in the management of moderate to severe pain and
3. as an antispasmodic agent in the treatment of renal and biliary colic.

Chemical   A synthetic phenylpiperidine derivative.

Presentation   As 50 mg tablets and a clear, colourless solution for injection containing 10/50 mg/ml of pethidine hydrochloride.

Main Actions   Analgesia and respiratory depression.

Mode of Action   Pethidine is an agonist at mu- and kappa-opioid receptors. Opioids appear to exert their effects by increasing intracellular calcium concentration, which in turn increases potassium conductance and hyperpolarisation of excitable cell membranes. The decrease in membrane excitability that results may decrease both pre- and post-synaptic responses.

Routes of Administration/Doses   The adult oral dose is 50–150 mg 4-hourly; the corresponding dose by the intramuscular route is 25–150 mg and by the intravenous route 25–100 mg. Pethidine may also be administered via the epidural route; a dose of 25 mg is usually employed. The drug acts within 15 minutes when administered orally and within 10 minutes when administered intramuscularly; the duration of action is 2–3 hours.

Effects
CVS   Pethidine causes orthostatic hypotension due to the combination of histamine release and alpha-adrenergic blockade that it produces. The drug also has a mild quinidine-like effect and anticholinergic properties, which may lead to the development of a tachycardia.
RS   The drug is a potent respiratory depressant, having a greater effect on tidal volume than on the respiratory rate. Pethidine obtunds the ventilatory response to both hypoxia and hypercapnia. Chest wall rigidity may occur with the use of the drug. It has little antitussive activity.
CNS   Pethidine is one-tenth as potent an analgesic as morphine. It appears to cause more euphoria and less nausea and vomiting than an equipotent dose of morphine. Miosis and corneal anaesthesia follow the use of the drug.
AS   In common with other opioids, pethidine decreases the rate of gastric emptying. The drug appears to cause a less marked increase in bile duct pressure and less depression of

98

intestinal activity (and therefore constipation) than equipotent doses of morphine.

GU The drug decreases ureteric tone; it may increase the amplitude of contractions of the pregnant uterus.

Metabolic/Other Pethidine increases ADH secretion and decreases adrenal steroid secretion.

Toxicity/Side Effects Respiratory depression, nausea and vomiting, hallucinations and dependence may complicate the use of pethidine. The drug evokes less histamine release than morphine.

Kinetics

Absorption The bioavailability when administered orally is 45–75%, due to a significant first-pass effect. The drug has a bioavailability of 100% when administered intramuscularly (into the deltoid muscle).

Distribution Pethidine is 49–67% protein-bound in the plasma; the V_D is 3.5–5.3 l/kg. The drug crosses the placenta; the mean cord blood concentration at delivery is 75–90% of the maternal venous concentration.

Metabolism Occurs in the liver by N-demethylation to norpethidine and by hydrolysis to pethidinic acid; norpethidine is further hydrolysed to norpethidinic acid. The acid metabolites are further conjugated prior to excretion. Norpethidine may accumulate in the presence of renal failure and has 50% the analgesic potency of the parent compound and marked convulsant properties.

Excretion 1–25% of the administered dose is excreted unchanged in the urine, dependent upon the urinary pH. Norpethidine is excreted in the urine; cumulation may occur in the presence of renal or hepatic impairment. The clearance is 12–22 ml/min/kg and the elimination half-life is 2.4–7 hours. The clearance is reduced by the co-administration of halothane.

Special Points Pethidine may precipitate a severe hypertensive episode in patients receiving MAOIs. The drug reduces the apparent MAC of co-administered volatile agents. By convention, pethidine is used in asthmatic patients although there is no published evidence that the drug causes bronchospasm less frequently than morphine in this group of patients.

Pethidine effectively inhibits post-anaesthetic shivering.

Phenelzine

Uses   Phenelzine is used in the treatment of:
1.   non-endogenous depression and
2.   phobic disorders.

Chemical   A substituted hydrazine.

Presentation   As tablets containing 15 mg of phenelzine sulphate.

Main Action   Antidepressant.

Mode of Action   Phenelzine is an irreversible inhibitor of mitochondrial monoamine oxidase, an enzyme involved in the metabolism of catecholamines and 5-hydroxytryptamine. It is assumed that the antidepressant activity of the drug is related to the increased concentration of monoamines in the central nervous system that results from the use of the drug.

Route of Administration/Dose   The adult oral dose is 15 mg 6–8 hourly; this is reduced once a satisfactory response has been obtained. The maximum inhibition of enzyme activity is achieved within a few days, but the antidepressant effect of the drug may take 3–4 weeks to become established.

Effects
CVS   The predominant effect of the drug is orthostatic hypotension; MAOIs were formerly used as antihypertensive agents.
CNS   Phenelzine is an effective antidepressant which may also produce stimulation of the central nervous system resulting in tremor and insomnia. The MAOIs suppress REM sleep very effectively.
AS   Constipation occurs commonly with the use of the drug – the mechanism of this effect is unknown.
Metabolic/Other   Inappropriate secretion of ADH has been reported in association with the use of phenelzine.

Toxicity/Side Effects   Disturbances of the central nervous system (including convulsions and peripheral neuropathy), anticholinergic side effects and hepatotoxicity may complicate the use of the drug. More importantly, a host of serious and potentially fatal interactions may occur between MAOIs and tyramine-containing substances, sympathomimetic agents and central nervous system depressants (*v.i.*).

Kinetics   Data are incomplete.

Absorption   Phenelzine is readily absorbed when administered orally.

Metabolism   80% of the dose is metabolised by oxidation and hydroxylation to phenylacetic acid and parahydroxy-phenylacetic acid. The drug may inhibit its own metabolism.

Excretion   Occurs predominantly in the urine as free and unconjugated aromatic forms of the drug.

Special Points   MAOIs demonstrate several important drug interactions:

1.   drugs such as pethidine, fentanyl, morphine and barbiturates whose action is terminated by oxidation have a more profound and prolonged effect in the presence of MAOIs; this is particularly marked in the case of pethidine. Marked hyperpyrexia, possibly due to 5-HT release, may also occur when pethidine is administered to a patient who is already receiving MAOIs

2.   indirectly – acting sympathomimetic agents (e.g. ephedrine) produce an exaggerated pressor response in the presence of co-administered MAOIs – severe hypertensive episodes (which are best treated with phentolamine) may result from this interaction.

3.   MAOIs markedly exaggerate the depressant effects of volatile anaesthetic agents on the blood pressure and central nervous system

4.   MAOIs inhibit plasma cholinesterase and may therefore prolong the duration of action of co-administered suxamethonium

5.   MAOIs may also potentiate the effects of antihypertensive and hypoglycaemic agents, anti-Parkinsonian drugs and local anaesthetics.

A period of two weeks is required to restore amine metabolism to normal after the cessation of administration of phenelzine. This is the recommended period that should elapse between discontinuation of MAOI therapy and elective surgery. Post-operative analgesia for patients who are still receiving MAOI therapy has been safely provided using chlorpromazine and codeine.

Phenoxybenzamine

Uses   Phenoxybenzamine is used in the treatment of:
1. hypertensive crises
2. Raynaud's phenomenon and
3. in the pre-operative preparation of patients due for the removal of a phaeochromocytoma.

Chemical   A tertiary amine which is a halo-alkylamine.

Presentation   As 10 mg tablets and a clear, colourless solution for injection containing 50 mg/ml of phenoxybenzamine hydrochloride.

Main Actions   Vasodilation (predominantly arterial).

Mode of Action   Phenoxybenzamine acts via a highly reactive carbonium ion derivative which binds covalently to alpha-adrenergic receptors to produce irreversible competitive alpha-blockade. The drug increases the rate of peripheral turnover of noradrenaline and the amount of noradrenaline released per impulse by blockade of pre-synaptic alpha-2 receptors. Haloalkylamines also inhibit the response to serotoninergic, histaminergic and cholinergic stimulation.

Routes of Administration/Doses   The adult dose by the oral route is 10–60 mg/day in divided doses. The corresponding dose by intravenous infusion (diluted in dextrose or saline) over 1 hour is 10–40 mg. After intravenous administration, the drug acts in 1 hour and has a duration of action of 3–4 days.

Effects
CVS   Phenoxybenzamine produces a decrease in the peripheral vascular resistance which leads to a decrease in the diastolic blood pressure and pronounced orthostatic hypotension. A reflex tachycardia and an increase in cardiac output follow the administration of the drug. Phenoxybenzamine inhibits catecholamine-induced cardiac dysrhythmias. The drug causes a shift of fluid from the interstitial to the vascular compartment due to vasodilation of pre- and post-capillary resistance vessels.
CNS   The drug decreases cerebral blood flow only if marked hypotension occurs. Motor excitability may follow the administration of phenoxybenzamine; however, sedation is the usual effect observed. Miosis occurs commonly.
AS   Phenoxybenzamine produces little change in gastrointestinal tone or splanchnic blood flow.
GU   The drug causes little alteration of renal blood flow; it decreases the motility of the non-pregnant uterus.

Toxicity/Side Effects   Dizziness, sedation, a dry mouth, paralytic ileus and impotence may result from the use of phenoxybenzamine. The drug is irritant if extravasation occurs.

Kinetics   Data are incomplete.

Absorption   Phenoxybenzamine is incompletely absorbed after oral administration; the bioavailability by this route is 20–30%.

Distribution   The drug is highly lipophilic.

Metabolism   Phenoxybenzamine is predominantly metabolised in the liver by deacetylation.

Excretion   Occurs via the urine and bile; the half-life is 24 hours.

Special Points   Systemic administration of the drug may lead to an increase in the systemic absorption of co-administered local anaesthetic agents. Phenoxybenzamine causes marked congestion of the nasal mucosa and this may make nasal instrumentation more traumatic if topical vasoconstrictors are not used.

Phentolamine

Uses   Phentolamine is used for:
1. the diagnosis and peri-operative management of patients with phaeochromocytoma
2. the acute treatment of hypertension occurring during anaesthesia and
3. the treatment of left ventricular failure complicating myocardial infarction.

Chemical   An imidazoline.

Presentation   As a clear solution for injection containing 10 mg/ml of phentolamine mesilate.

Main Actions   Hypotension, positive inotropism and chronotropism.

Mode of Action   Phentolamine acts by transient competitive alpha-adrenergic blockade (it is 3–5 times as active at alpha-1 as at alpha-2 receptors); it also has some beta-adrenergic agonist and anti-serotoninergic activity.

Routes of Administration/Doses   The adult intramuscular dose for the control of paroxysmal hypertension is 5–10 mg; the drug may also be administered by intravenous infusion (diluted in dextrose or saline) at the rate of 0.1–0.2 mg/min.

Effects
CVS   Phentolamine causes a marked reduction in the systemic vascular resistance, producing a decrease in blood pressure and a reflex tachycardia. The drug has a positive inotropic action, which is probably an indirect effect due to alpha-2 blockade leading to noradrenaline release. The coronary blood flow increases; the drug also has class I antiarrhythmic effects. In patients with heart failure, phentolamine causes an increase in the heart rate and cardiac output, with a concomitant decrease in the pulmonary arterial pressure, systemic vascular resistance and left ventricular end-diastolic pressure.
RS   The drug increases the vital capacity, FEV_1 and maximum breathing capacity in normal subjects, and prevents histamine-induced bronchoconstriction. Respiratory tract secretions are increased by the drug. Phentolamine is a pulmonary arterial vasodilator.
AS   The drug increases salivation, gastric acid and pepsin secretion and gastrointestinal motility.
Metabolic/Other   The drug increases insulin secretion.

Toxicity/Side Effects   Phentolamine is generally well tolerated, but may cause orthostatic hypotension, dizziness, abdominal discomfort and diarrhoea. Cardiovascular collapse and death have followed the administration of phentolamine when it is used as a diagnostic test for phaeochromocytoma.

Kinetics   Data are incomplete.

Absorption   The bioavailability is 20% when administered orally.

Excretion   10% of the dose is excreted in the urine unchanged. The plasma half-life is 10–15 minutes.

Special Points   Phentolamine causes marked congestion of the nasal mucosa and this may make nasal instrumentation more traumatic if topical vasoconstrictors are not used.

Phenytoin

Uses Phenytoin is used:
1. in the prophylaxis and treatment of generalised tonic-clonic and partial epilepsies and in the treatment of
2. fast atrial and ventricular dysrhythmias resulting from digoxin toxicity and
3. trigeminal neuralgia.

Chemical A hydantoin derivative.

Presentation As 25/50/100/300 mg capsules, a syrup containing 6 mg/ml and as a clear, colourless solution for injection containing 50 mg/ml of phenytoin sodium.

Main Actions Anticonvulsant and antiarrhythmic.

Mode of Action Phenytoin has membrane stabilising activity and slows inwards sodium and calcium ion flux during depolarisation in excitable tissue; it also delays outwards potassium ion flux. There appears to be a high-affinity binding site within the central nervous system for phenytoin which suggests the existence of an endogenous ligand.

Routes of Administration/Doses The adult oral dose is 200–600 mg/day; a small dose should be used initially and gradually increased thereafter. The corresponding intramuscular dose is 100–200 mg 4-hourly for 48–72 hours, decreasing to 300 mg daily. The intravenous loading dose for the management of epilepsy is 10–15 mg/kg (administered slowly), followed by a maintenance dose of 100 mg 6–8-hourly. When used in the treatment of cardiac dysrhythmias, the corresponding intravenous dose is 3.5 mg/kg. The therapeutic range is 10–20 mg/l.

Effects
CVS Phenytoin exhibits class I antiarrhythmic properties and enhances atrio-ventricular nodal conduction. Hypotension may complicate rapid intravenous administration of the drug; complete heart block, ventricular fibrillation and asystole have also been reported under these circumstances.
CNS 80% of newly diagnosed epileptics can be controlled with phenytoin monotherapy. The drug acts as an ariticovulsant by stabilising rather than raising the seizure threshold and by preventing the spread of seizure activity rather than by abolishing a primary discharging focus.
Metabolic/Other Hyperglycaemia, hypocalcaemia and alterations in liver function tests have been described consequent to phenytoin therapy. The drug suppresses ADH secretion.

Toxicity/Side Effects Phenytoin has both idiosyncratic and concentration-dependent side effects. The idiosyncratic side effects include acne, gum hyperplasia, hirsutism, coarsened facies, folate-dependent megaloblastic anaemia and other blood dyscrasias, osteomalacia, erythroderma, lymphadenopathy, systemic lupus erythematosus, hepatotoxicity and allergic phenomena. The concentration-dependent side effects include nausea and vomiting, drowsiness, behavioural disturbances, tremor, ataxia, nystagmus, paradoxical seizures, peripheral neuropathy and cerebellar damage. The drug is irritant if extravasation occurs when given intravenously and may cause muscular damage when administered intramuscularly.

Kinetics

Absorption   Absorption is very slow by both the intramuscular and oral routes. The oral bioavailability is 85–95%.

Distribution   Phenytoin is 90–93% protein-bound in the plasma; the V_D is 0.5–0.7 l/kg.

Metabolism   There is a large genetic variation in the rate of metabolism of phenytoin, which occurs in the liver predominantly to a hydroxylated derivative which is subsequently conjugated to glucuronide. Phenytoin exhibits zero-order elimination kinetics just above the therapeutic range; the implication of this is that the dose required to produce a plasma concentration within the therapeutic range is close to that which will produce toxicity.

Excretion   70–80% of the dose is excreted in the urine by active tubular secretion as the major metabolite; <5% is excreted unchanged. The clearance is 5.5–9.5 ml/kg/day and the elimination half-life is 9–22 hours in the first-order kinetics range; the latter increases at higher dose ranges when the capacity of the hepatic mono-oxygenase system becomes saturated. The dose of phenytoin should be reduced in the presence of hepatic impairment, but renal impairment requires little alteration of dosage (despite the fact that the free fraction of the drug increases in the presence of uraemia, an increase in the clearance and V_D tend to offset this).

Special Points   Phenytoin is a potent enzyme inducer and demonstrates a plethora of drug interactions, amongst which the most important are the precipitation of phenytoin toxicity by metronidazole and isoniazid and a reduced effectiveness of benzodiazepines, pethidine and warfarin caused by the co-administration of phenytoin. The drug may also decrease the MAC of volatile agents and enhance the central nervous system toxicity of local anaesthetics; it appears to increase the dose requirements of all the non-depolarising relaxants (with the exception of atracurium) by 60–80%.

The parenteral preparation of phenytoin precipitates in the presence of most crystalloid solutions.

The drug is not removed by dialysis.

Piperacillin

Uses   Piperacillin is used in the treatment of:
1. urinary and respiratory tract infections
2. intra-abdominal and biliary tract sepsis
3. gynaecological and obstetric infections
4. infections of skin, soft tissue, bone and joints
5. septicaemia
6. meningitis and for
7. peri-operative prophylaxis.

Chemical   A semi-synthetic penicillin.

Presentation   In vials containing 1/2 g and infusion bottles containing 4 g of piperacillin sodium. A fixed dose combination with tazobactam is also available.

Main Actions   Piperacillin is a bactericidal broad spectrum antibiotic that is effective against many beta-lactamase-producing organisms. *In vitro*, it shows activity against the Gram-negative organisms *Escherichia coli, Haemophilus influenzae* and *Klebsiella, Neisseria, Proteus, Shigella* and *Serratia* sp.; anaerobes including *Bacteroides* and *Clostridium* sp. and the Gram-positive enterococci, *Staphylococcus* and *Streptococcus* sp. It is particularly effective against *Pseudomonas,* indole-positive *Proteus, Streptococcus faecalis* and *Serratia marcescens.*

Mode of Action   Piperacillin binds to cell wall penicillin-binding proteins (PBPs) and inhibits their activity; specifically, it affects PBP 1A/B which are involved in the cross-linking of cell wall peptidoglycans, PBP 2 which is involved in the maintenance of the rod shape and PBP 3 which is involved in septal synthesis.

Routes of Administration/Doses   The adult intravenous dose is 4 g 6–8 hourly (each gram should be infused over 3–5 minutes) and the intramuscular dose 2 g 6–8 hourly.

Effects
Metabolic/Other   Piperacillin has a lower sodium content than other disodium penicillins and causes less fluid and electrolyte derangements; serum potassium levels may decrease after the administration of the drug.

Toxicity/Side Effects   Gastrointestinal upsets, abnormalities of liver function tests, allergic reactions and transient leucopenia and neutropenia may complicate the use of the drug. Deterioration in renal function has been reported in patients with pre-existent severe renal impairment treated with piperacillin.

Kinetics

Absorption Piperacillin is poorly absorbed when administered orally and is hydrolysed by gastric acids.

Distribution The drug is 16% protein-bound in the plasma; the V_D is 0.32 l/kg. High concentrations are found in most tissues and body fluids.

Metabolism Piperacillin is not metabolised in man.

Excretion 20% is excreted in the bile; the remainder is excreted in the urine by glomerular filtration and tubular secretion. The elimination half-life is 36–72 minutes.

Special Points The dose of piperacillin should be reduced in the presence of renal impairment; the drug is 30–50% removed by haemodialysis.

Polygeline

Uses Polygeline is used:
1. for plasma volume replacement in haemorrhage, burns or excessive fluid and electrolyte loss
2. for extracorporeal circulation, isolated organ perfusion and plasma exchange and
3. as a carrier solution for insulin.

Chemical Polygeline is a polypeptide produced by the thermal degradation of bovine gelatin – the hydrolysate thus formed consists of small polypeptides of molecular weight 12 000–15 000 daltons. These are then cross-linked via urea bridges to yield molecules with an average molecular weight of 35 000 and subsequently dissolved in water. The ionic composition is then adjusted to yield the formulation described below.

Presentation Polygeline is presented in 500 ml plastic bottles containing a sterile, pyrogen-free, straw-coloured solution of pH 7.2. Each litre contains 35 g of polygeline, 145 mmol of sodium and chloride ions, 5.1 mmol of potassium ions and 6.25 mmol of calcium ions.

Main Action Plasma volume expansion.

Mode of Action Polygeline equilibrates throughout the body (28% in circulating blood, 27–31% in the interstitial space and 40–46% in urine) to restore the haemodynamic status after a period of hypovolaemia.

Route of Administration/Dose Polygeline is administered intravenously as required to restore the circulating volume: it should not be used to restore greater than 25% of the total circulating blood volume.

Effects
CVS The haemodynamic effects of polygeline are proportional to the prevailing volaemic status.
GU Renal perfusion is restored towards normal in hypovolaemic subjects transfused with the colloid; in addition, polygeline has an osmotic diuretic effect.
Metabolic/Other Polygeline has no effect on the blood sugar concentration, and no specific effect on coagulation or fibrinolysis.

Toxicity/Side Effects A degree of histamine release occurs in 1 in 1000 patients who receive the colloid; since the preparation is non-immunogenic, it is assumed that this is an anaphylactoid response. Severe, life-threatening reactions are very rare.

Kinetics

Distribution The distribution of polygeline has been described earlier; the V_D is 9–13 l.

Metabolism *In vitro* studies suggest that polygeline is degraded by proteolytic enzymes to smaller peptides and amino acids.

Excretion 74% is excreted in the urine within 4 days; about 10% is excreted in the faeces. Excretion is complete after 12 days. Two fractions are recognised – 30% consists of a small molecular weight fraction which is rapidly excreted (with an elimination half-life of 0.2–0.4 hours in animals) and the remaining 70% consists of a larger molecular weight fraction which is excreted with an elimination half-life of 8.4 hours in man.

Special Points Polygeline contains ionic calcium and may thus enhance the toxicity of digoxin administered concurrently and may also cause coagulation of citraced blood (with which it should not be mixed). It has no effect on blood cross-matching.

The use of polygeline is not recommended as a prophylactic measure against the occurrence of hypotension in patients undergoing spinal or epidural anaesthesia.

Prazosin

Uses   Prazosin is used in the treatment of:
1. hypertension
2. Raynaud's phenomenon and may be of use in the treatment of
3. congestive cardiac failure
4. aortic and mitral regurgitation
5. phaeochromocytoma and
6. bladder neck obstruction.

Chemical   A quinazoline derivative.

Presentation   As tablets containing 0.5/1/2/5 mg of prazosin hydrochloride.

Main Actions   Arterial and venous vasodilation.

Mode of Action   Prazosin is a highly selective competitive antagonist of alpha-1 (post-synaptic) adrenoceptors, thereby causing relaxation of vascular smooth muscle.

Routes of Administration/Doses   The adult dose is 1 mg 8–12 hourly (introduced cautiously) increased to a total of 20 mg daily.

Effects
CVS   Prazosin dilates coronary arteries, peripheral arterioles and veins, leading to a decrease in the pulmonary and systemic vascular resistance and blood pressure. Relatively little reflex tachycardia occurs; the drug may have a direct negative chronotropic effect on the sinus node. The cardiac output may increase in patients with heart failure who receive the drug.
RS   Prazosin produces clinically insignificant bronchodilatation in some asthmatic subjects.
GU   Prazosin has little effect on the renal blood flow or glomerular filtration rate. The drug causes relaxation of the bladder trigone and sphincter muscle.
Metabolic/Other   Prazosin may cause a significant increase in the plasma noradrenaline concentration; it has little effect on plasma renin activity.

Toxicity/Side Effects   Prazosin is generally well tolerated. Postural hypotension, drowsiness, fatigue, nausea and urinary urgency may occur. The 'first-dose phenomenon' consists of dizziness and faintness, possibly accompanied by palpitations, occurring as a result of profound hypotension, bradycardia and decreased venous return.

Kinetics

Absorption   The oral absorption is variable; the bioavailability by this route is 43–62%.

Distribution   Prazosin is 92% protein-bound in the plasma, predominantly to an acid glycoprotein. The V_D is 0.5–0.89 l/kg.

Metabolism   Occurs via dealkylation in the liver – the metabolites are active.

Excretion   Excretion occurs predominantly in the bile and faeces; less than 10% is excreted unchanged. The clearance is 3.5–4 ml/kg/min and the elimination half-life is 2.5–2.9 hours.

Special Points   False positive results may occur in patients undergoing screening tests for phaeochromocytoma. An additive hypocensive effect should be expected with co-administered volatile anaesthetic agents.

The drug is not removed by dialysis.

Prednisolone

Uses   Prednisolone is used:
1. as replacement therapy in adrenocortical deficiency states and in the treatment of
2. allergy and anaphylaxis
3. hypercalcaemia
4. asthma
5. a panoply of autoimmune disorders
6. some forms of red eye and
7. in leukaemia chemotherapy regimes and
8. for immunosupression after organ transplantation.

Chemical   A synthetic glucocorticosteroid.

Presentation   As 1/2.5/5/20 mg tablets of prednisolone, a solution for injection containing 25 mg/ml of prednisolone acetate and as eye/ear drops and retention enemas.

Main Action   Anti-inflammatory.

Mode of Action   Corticosteroids act by controlling the rate of protein synthesis; they react with cytoplasmic receptors to form a complex which directly influences the rate of RNA transcription. This directs the synthesis of lipocortins.

Routes of Administration/Doses   The adult oral dose is 5–60 mg/day in divided doses, using the lowest dose that is effective and on alternate days if possible to limit the development of side effects. The intramuscular or intra-articular dose is 25–100 mg once or twice weekly.

Effects
CVS   In the absence of corticosteroids vascular permeability increases, small blood vessels demonstrate an inadequate motor response and cardiac output decreases. Steroids have a positive effect on myocardial contractility and cause vasoconstriction by increasing the number of alpha-1 adrenoreceptors and beta-adrenoreceptors and stimulating their function.
CNS   Corticosteroids increase the excitability of the central nervous system; the absence of glucocorticoid leads to apathy, depression and irritability.
AS   Prednisolone increases the likelihood of peptic ulcer disease. It decreases the gastrointestinal absorption of calcium.
GU   Prednisolone has weak mineralocorticoid effects and produces sodium retention and increased potassium excretion; the urinary excretion of calcium is also increased by the drug. The drug increases the glomerular filtration rate and stimulates tubular secretory activity.

Metabolic/Other Prednisolone exerts profound effects on carbohydrate, protein and lipid metabolism. Glucocorticoids stimulate gluconeogenesis and inhibit the peripheral utilisation of glucose; they cause a redistribution of body fat, enhance lipolysis and also reduce the conversion of amino acids to protein. Prednisolone is a potent anti-inflammatory agent which inhibits all stages of the inflammatory process by inhibiting neutrophil and macrophage recruitment, blocking the effect of lymphokines and inhibiting the formation of plasminogen activator. Corticosteroids increase red blood cell, neutrophil and haemoglobin concentrations, whilst depressing other white cell lines and the activity of lymphoid tissue.

Toxicity/Side Effects Consist of an acute withdrawal syndrome and a syndrome (Cushing's) produced by prolonged use of excessive quantities of the drug. Cushing's syndrome is characterised by growth arrest, a characteristic appearance consisting of central obesity, a moon face and buffalo hump, striae, acne, hirsutism, skin and capillary fragility together with the following metabolic derangements: altered glucose tolerance, fluid retention, a hypokalaemic alkalosis and osteoporosis. A proximal myopathy, cataracts, mania and an increased susceptibility to peptic ulcer disease may also complicate the use of the drug.

Kinetics

Absorption Prednisolone is rapidly and completely absorbed when administered orally or rectally; the bioavailability by either route is 80–100%.

Distribution The drug is reversibly bound in the plasma to albumin and a specific corticosteroid binding globulin; the drug is 80–90% protein-bound at low concentrations but only 60–70% protein-bound at higher concentrations. The V_D is 0.35–0.7 l/kg according to the dose.

Metabolism Occurs in the liver by hydroxylation with subsequent conjugation.

Excretion 11–14% of the dose is excreted unchanged in the urine. The clearance is dose-dependent and ranges from 170–200 ml/min; the elimination half-life is 2.6–5 hours.

Special Points Prednisone and prednisolone are metabolically interconvertible; only the latter is active. The conversion of prednisone to prednisolone is rapid and extensive and occurs as a first-pass effect in the liver. Prednisolone is 4 times as potent as hydrocortisone and 6 times less potent than dexamethasone. It has been recommended that peri-operative

Prednisolone

steroid cover be given:

1. to patients who have received steroid replacement therapy for >2 weeks prior to surgery or for >1 month in the year prior to surgery and
2. to patients undergoing pituitary or adrenal surgery. Glucocorticoids antagonise the effects of anticholinesterase drugs.

Prilocaine

Uses   Prilocaine is used as a local anaesthetic.

Chemical   A secondary amine which is an amide derivative of toluidine.

Presentation   As a clear, colourless 0.5/1/2/4% solution for injection of prilocaine hydrochloride and a 3% solution with 0.03 IU of felypressin per ml.

Main Action   Local anaesthetic.

Mode of Action   Local anaesthetics diffuse in their uncharged base form through neural sheaths and the axonal membrane to the internal surface of cell membrane sodium ion channels; here they combine with hydrogen ions to form a cationic species which enters the internal opening of the sodium ion channel and combines with a receptor. This produces blockade of the sodium ion channel, thereby decreasing sodium ion conductance and preventing depolarisation of the cell membrane.

Routes of Administration/Doses   Prilocaine may be administered topically, by infiltration, or epidurally; the toxic dose of prilocaine is 6 mg/kg (8 mg/kg with felypressin). Prilocaine has a duration of action 1.5 times that of lignocaine.

Effects
CVS   Prilocaine has few haemodynamic effects when used in low doses, except to cause a slight increase in the systemic vascular resistance leading to a mild increase in the blood pressure. In toxic concentrations, the drug decreases peripheral vascular resistance and myocardial contractility, producing hypotension and possibly cardiovascular collapse.
RS   The drug causes bronchodilatation at subtoxic concentrations. Respiratory depression occurs in the toxic dose range.
CNS   The principal effect of prilocaine is reversible neural blockade; this leads to a characteristically biphasic effect in the central nervous system. Initially, excitation (lightheadedness, dizziness, visual and auditory disturbances and fitting) occurs, due to the blockade of inhibitory pathways in the cortex; with increasing doses, depression of both facilitatory and inhibitory pathways occur, leading to central nervous system depression (drowsiness, disorientation and coma). Local anaesthetic agents block neuromuscular transmission when administered intra-arterially; it is thought that a complex of neurotransmitter, receptor and local anaesthetic is formed which has negligible conductance.
AS   Local anaesthetics depress contraction of the intact bowel.

Toxicity/Side Effects Prilocaine is intrinsically less toxic than lignocaine. Allergic reactions to the amide-type local anaesthetic agents are extremely rare. The side effects are predominantly correlated with excessive plasma concentrations of the drug. Methaemoglobinaemia may occur if doses in excess of 600 mg are administered to an adult (*v.i.*).

Kinetics Data are incomplete.

Absorption The absorption of local anaesthetic agents is related to:

1. the site of injection (intercostal > epidural > brachial plexus > subcutaneous)
2. the dose – a linear relationship exists between the total dose and the peak blood concentrations achieved and
3. the presence of vasoconstrictors, which delay absorption.

Distribution Prilocaine is 55% protein-bound in the plasma, predominantly to alpha-1 acid glycoprotein.

Metabolism Prilocaine is rapidly metabolised in the liver, initially to O-toluidine which is in turn metabolised to 4- and 6-hydroxytoluidine. Some metabolism occurs also in the lung and kidney. Excessive plasma concentrations of O-toluidine may lead to the development of methaemoglobinaemia, which responds to the intravenous administration of 1–2 mg/kg of methylene blue.

Excretion Occurs as inactive metabolites in the urine, <1% unchanged.

Special Points The onset and duration of conduction blockade is related to the pKa, lipid solubility and extent of protein binding of the drug. A low pKa and a high lipid solubility are associated with a rapid onset time; a high degree of protein binding is associated with a long duration of action. The pKa of prilocaine is 7.9 and the heptane:buffer partition coefficient is 0.9.

Local anaesthetic agents significantly increase the duration of action of both depolarising and non-depolarising relaxants.

EMLA (Eutectic Mixture of Local Anaesthetics) is a white cream used to provide topical anaesthesia prior to venepuncture, and has also been used to provide anaesthesia for split-skin grafting. It contains 2.5% lignocaine and 2.5% prilocaine in an oil–water emulsion. When applied topically under an occlusive dressing, local anaesthesia is achieved after 1–2 hours and lasts for up to 5 hours. The preparation causes temporary blanching and oedema of the skin; detectable methaemoglobinaemia may also occur.

Prochlorperazine

Uses   Prochlorperazine is used in the treatment of:
1. nausea and vomiting
2. vertigo
3. psychotic states, including mania and schizophrenia and
4. in premedication.

Chemical   A phenothiazine of the piperazine subclass.

Presentation   As tablets containing 3/5/25 mg, suppositories containing 5/25 mg, as a clear, colourless solution for injection containing 12.5 mg/ml of prochlorperazine maleate, and as a syrup containing 1 mg/ml of prochlorperazine mesylate.

Main Actions   Antiemetic.

Mode of Action   The antiemetic and neuroleptic effects of the drug appear to be mediated by central dopaminergic (D_2-) blockade leading to an increased threshold for vomiting at the chemoreceptor trigger zone; in higher doses, prochlorperazine appears to have an inhibitory effect at the vomiting centre.

Routes of Administration/Doses   The adult dose is 5–20 mg 8–12 hourly and the corresponding intramuscular dose is 12.5 mg 6-hourly.

Effects
CVS   Prochlorperazine may cause orthostatic hypotension secondary to alpha-adrenergic blockade. ECG changes, including an increased Q-T interval, ST depression and T- and U-wave changes, may also occur.
RS   The drug may cause mild respiratory depression.
CNS   Prochlorperazine has neuroleptic properties but appears to be less soporific than perphenazine.
AS   Lower oesophageal tone is increased by the drug.
Metabolic/Other   In common with other phenothiazines, prochlorperazine has antiadrenergic, anti-inflammatory, antipruritic, anticholinergic and antihistaminergic effects. The drug may also cause hyperprolactinaemia.

Toxicity/Side Effects   Prochlorperazine may cause extrapyramidal reactions, jaundice, leucopenia and rashes. The neuroleptic malignant syndrome (a complex of symptoms that include catatonia, cardiovascular lability, hyperthermia and myoglobinaemia) which has a mortality in excess of 10% has been reported in association with the use of the drug.

Kinetics   Data are incomplete.

Absorption   The drug is slowly absorbed when administered orally; the bioavailability is 0–16% by this route.

Distribution   The degree of protein-binding of prochlorperazine is unknown; the V_D is 20–22 l/kg.

Metabolism   Prochlorperazine undergoes significant first-pass metabolism in the liver; its metabolic pathways remain poorly elucidated. Metabolism may occur by S-oxidation to a sulphoxide.

Special Points   Prochlorperazine is not removed by haemodialysis.

Promethazine

Uses Promethazine is used in the treatment of:
1. nausea and vomiting (including motion sickness)
2. allergic reactions
3. pruritus and for
4. sedation in children.

Chemical A phenothiazine.

Presentation As 10/25 mg tablets, an elixir containing 1 mg/ml and a clear, colourless solution for injection containing 25 mg/ml of promethazine hydrochloride.

Main Actions Antihistaminergic, sedative and antiemetic.

Mode of Action Promethazine acts primarily as a reversible competitive antagonist at H1 histaminergic receptors; it also has some anticholinergic, antiserotoninergic and antidopaminergic activity.

Routes of Administration/Doses The adult oral dose is 20–75 mg daily in divided doses; the corresponding intramuscular and intravenous dose is 25–50 mg. The drug acts within 15 minutes and has a duration of action of 8–20 hours.

Effects
CVS When normal therapeutic doses are used, promethazine has no significant cardiovascular effects. Rapid intravenous administration may cause transient hypotension.
RS The drug causes bronchodilatation, a reduction in respiratory tract secretions and has antitussive properties.
CNS Promethazine is a potent sedative and anxiolytic; it also has a slight antanalgesic effect. It reduces motion sickness by suppression of vestibular end-organ receptors and by an inhibitory action at the chemoreceptor trigger zone. The drug has local anaesthetic properties.
AS Promethazine decreases the tone of the lower oesophageal sphincter.

Toxicity/Side Effects The drug exhibits predictable anticholinergic side effects and may produce extra-pyramidal reactions when used in high doses. Jaundice, photosensitivity, excitatory phenomena, gastrointestinal and haemopoietic disturbances may complicate the use of promethazine.

Kinetics

Absorption Promethazine is well absorbed when administered orally, but undergoes an extensive first-pass metabolism.

Distribution The drug is 93% protein-bound in the plasma; the V_D is 2.5 l/kg.

Metabolism Promethazine is metabolised in the liver by sulphoxidation and N-dealkylation.

Excretion Occurs predominantly in the urine, 2% unchanged. The clearance is 1.41 l/min and the elimination half-life is 7.5–10 hours.

Special Points The depressant effects of the drug on the central nervous system are additive with those produced by anaesthetic agents.

Promethazine is not removed by haemodialysis.

Propofol

Uses Propofol is used:
1. for the induction and maintenance of general anaesthesia
2. for sedation during intensive care and regional anaesthesia and has been used
3. in the treatment of refractory nausea and vomiting in patients receiving chemotherapy and
4. in the treatment of status epilepticus.

Chemical Propofol is 2,6-diisopropylphenol; a phenol derivative.

Presentation As a white oil-in-water emulsion containing 1% or 2% w/v of propofol in soybean oil, purified egg phosphatide, and sodium hydroxide.

Main Action Hypnotic.

Mode of Action The mode of action of propofol is unclear. It potentiates the inhibitory transmitters glycine and GABA which enhance spinal inhibition during anaesthesia.

Routes of Administration/Doses Propofol is administered intravenously in a bolus dose of 1.5–2.5 mg/kg for induction and as an infusion of 4–12 mg/kg/hour for maintenance of anaesthesia. For children, the induction dose should be increased by 50% and the maintenance infusion by 25–50%. Consciousness is lost in about 30 seconds and waking occurs about 10 minutes after a single dose. Plasma concentrations of 2–6 µg/ml and 0.5–1.5 µg/ml are associated with hypnosis and sedation respectively.

Effects
CVS Propofol produces a 15–25% decrease in the blood pressure and systemic vascular resistance without a compensatory increase in heart rate; the cardiac output decreases by 20%. In fit patients, the drug attenuates the haemodynamic response to laryngoscopy. Vasodilation occurs secondary to propofol-stimulated production and release of nitric oxide. Profound bradycardia and asystole may complicate the use of the drug.
RS Bolus administration of propofol produces apnoea of variable duration and suppression of laryngeal reflexes. Infusion of the drug produces a decrease in tidal volume, tachypnoea and a depressed ventilatory response to hypercarbia and hypoxia. Propofol causes bronchodilation possibly via a direct effect on bronchial smooth muscle. The drug does not increase intrapulmonary shunting and may preserve the mechanism of hypoxic pulmonary vasoconstriction.
CNS Propofol produces a smooth, rapid induction with rapid and clear-headed recovery. Intracranial pressure, cerebral

perfusion pressure and cerebral oxygen consumption all decrease following administration of the drug. In animal models, propofol exhibits anticonvulsant properties. There is no evidence that the drug produces epileptiform activity in non-epileptic patients. Involuntary movements after propofol are not accompanied by seizure activity on EEG recordings.

AS Propofol appears to possess intrinsic antiemetic properties which may be mediated by antagonism of dopamine D_2 receptors.

GU In animals, propofol causes a reduction in the excretion of sodium ions.

Metabolic/Other Long-term use of propofol infusions may result in hypertriglyceridaemia. The 1% preparation has a calorific value of 1 Cal/ml. Clinically significant impairment of adrenal steroidogenesis does not occur. Propofol is a free-radical scavenger.

Toxicity/Side Effects Pain on injection occurs in up to 28% of subjects. The incidence may be reduced by addition of lignocaine, cooling the drug and the use of large veins. There are case reports of epileptiform movements, facial parasthesiae and bradycardia following the administration of propofol, although the incidence of allergic phenomena is low. The use of propofol appears to be safe in patients susceptible to porphyria (although urinary porphyrin concentrations may increase) and malignant hyperpyrexia. There are reports of neurological sequelae and increased mortality complicating long-term use of propofol for sedation of children receiving intensive therapy. The quinol metabolites may occasionally cause green discoloration of the urine and green hair.

Kinetics

Distribution Propofol is 97% protein-bound in the plasma; the V_D is 700–1500 l. The distribution half-life is 1.3–4.1 minutes, resulting in a brief duration of anaesthesia following bolus administration of the drug.

Metabolism Propofol is rapidly metabolised in the liver, primarily to inactive glucuronide (49–73%), and sulphate and glucuronide conjugates of the hydroxylated metabolite via cytochrome P-450. Interpatient variability determines the ratio between glucuronide and hydroxylated pathway. Extrahepatic mechanisms may contribute to the metabolism of the drug. Renal and hepatic disease have no clinically significant effect on the metabolism of propofol.

Excretion The metabolites are excreted in the urine; 0.3% is excreted unchanged. The clearance is 18.8–40.3 ml/kg/min and the elimination half-life is 9.3–69.3 minutes. The clearance is decreased in the presence of renal failure. Under normal conditions, propofol is non-cumulative.

Propofol

Special Points Propofol may increase the energy required for successful cardioversion. The drug causes shortened duration of seizure activity during electroconvulsive therapy, although it does not decrease the efficacy of the treatment. Propofol is physically incompatible with atracurium. Aqueous emulsions of the drug support both bacterial and fungal growth.

Propranolol

Uses   Propranolol is used in the treatment of:
1. hypertension
2. angina
3. a variety of cardiac tachydysrhythmias
4. essential tremor and in the adjunctive management of
5. anxiety
6. thyrotoxicosis
7. hypertrophic obstructive cardiomyopathy
8. phaeochromocytoma and in the prophylaxis of
9. recurrence of myocardial infarction and
10. migraine.

Chemical   An aromatic amine.

Presentation   As tablets containing 10/40/80/160 mg, and as a clear solution for injection containing 1 mg/ml of propranolol hydrochloride.

Main Actions   Negative inotropism and chronotropism.

Mode of Action   Propranolol acts by competitive antagonism of beta-1 and beta-2 adrenoceptors; it has no intrinsic sympathomimetic activity. It also exerts a membrane stabilising effect when used in very high doses by the inhibition of sodium ion currents.

Routes of Administration/Doses   The adult oral dose is 30–320 mg/day in 2–3 divided doses, according to the condition requiring treatment. The corresponding dose by the intravenous route is 1–10 mg, titrated according to response.

Effects
CVS   Propranolol is negatively inotropic and chronotropic and leads to a decrease in myocardial oxygen consumption; the mechanism of the drug's antihypertensive action remains poorly defined. Blockade of beta-2 adrenoceptors produces an increase in the peripheral vascular resistance.
RS   Propranolol causes a decrease in FEV_1 by increasing airways resistance; it also attenuates the ventilatory response to hypercapnia.
CNS   The drug crosses the blood–brain barrier; its central effects may be involved in the mechanism of the drug's antihypertensive action. Propranolol diminishes physiological tremor and decreases intraocular pressure.
GU   Propranolol decreases uterine tone, especially during pregnancy.
Metabolic/Other   The drug decreases plasma renin activity and suppresses aldosterone release. Propranolol causes a decrease in the plasma free fatty acid concentration and may

also cause hypoglycaemia due to blockade of gluconeogenesis. The drug increases total body sodium concentration and thus the extracellular fluid volume.

Toxicity/Side Effects The side effects of propranolol are predictable manifestations of non-specific beta-adrenergic blockade. The drug may thus precipitate heart failure or heart block, exacerbate peripheral vascular disease, lead to bronchospasm, sleep disturbances and nightmares, mask the symptoms of hypoglycaemia and cause impaired exercise tolerance.

Kinetics

Absorption 90% of an oral dose of propranolol is absorbed; the bioavailability is 30–35% due to an extensive first-pass metabolism.

Distribution The drug is 90–96% protein-bound in the plasma, predominantly to alpha-1 acid glycoprotein; the V_D is 3.6 l/kg.

Metabolism Propranolol undergoes extensive hepatic metabolism by oxidative deamination and dealkylation with subsequent glucuronidarion; the 4-hydroxy metabolite is active.

Excretion Occurs via the urine; less than 1% of the dose is excreted unchanged. The clearance is 0.5–1.2 l/min and the elimination half-life is 2–4 hours. The dose should be reduced in the presence of hepatic failure; no alteration in dose is necessary in the presence of renal impairment.

Special Points Beta-adrenergic blockade should be continued throughout the peri-operative period; abrupt withdrawal of propranolol may precipitate angina, ventricular dysrhythmias, myocardial infarction and sudden death. The co-administration of propranolol and non-depolarising relaxants may lead to a slight potentiation of the latter.

The drug is not removed by dialysis.

Protamine

Uses Protamine is used:
1. to neutralise the anticoagulant effects of heparin and
2. to prolong the effects of insulin.

Chemical A purified mixture of low-molecular-weight cationic proteins prepared from fish sperm.

Presentation As a clear, colourless solution for injection containing 10 mg/ml of protamine sulphate.

Main Actions Neutralisation of the anticoagulant effect of heparin; in high doses, protamine has a weak intrinsic anticoagulant effect.

Mode of Action Both *in vitro* and *in vivo*, the strongly basic compound protamine complexes with the strongly acidic compound heparin to form a stable salt – this complex is inactive. The intrinsic anticoagulant effect of the drug appears to be due to the inhibition of the formation and activity of thromboplastin.

Route of Administration/Dose Protamine is administered by slow intravenous injection; the dose should be adjusted according to the amount of heparin that is to be neutralised, the time that has elapsed since the administration of heparin and the Activated Coagulation Time (ACT). 1 mg of protamine will neutralise 100 units of heparin. A maximum adult dose of 50 mg of the drug should be administered in any 10-minute period.

Effects
CVS Protamine is a myocardial depressant and may cause bradycardia and hypotension secondary to complement activation and leukotriene release. The pulmonary artery pressure may increase, leading to an impairment of right ventricular output.

Toxicity/Side Effects Rapid intravenous administration of protamine may be complicated by acute hypotension, bradycardia, dyspnoea and flushing. Anaphylactoid reactions may also occur; antibodies to human protamine often develop in vasecromised males and may predispose to hypersensitivity phenomena.

Kinetics Data are incomplete.

Metabolism The metabolic fate of the protamine heparin complex has not been well elucidated; it may undergo partial degradation, thereby freeing heparin.

Ranitidine

Uses Ranitidine is used in the treatment of:
1. peptic ulcer disease
2. reflux oesophagitis
3. the Zollinger-Ellison syndrome and
4. for the prevention of stress ulceration in critically ill patients and
5. prior to general anaesthesia in patients at risk of acid aspiration, especially during pregnancy and labour.

Chemical A furan derivative.

Presentation As a clear solution for intravenous or intramuscular injection containing 25 mg/ml, as 150/300 mg tablets and as a syrup containing 15 mg/ml of ranitidine hydrochloride.

Main Actions Inhibition of gastric acid secretion.

Mode of Action Ranitidine acts via competitive blockade of histaminergic H2 receptors. Histamine appears to be necessary to potentiate the action of gastrin and acetylcholine on the gastric parietal cell, as well as acting directly as a secretogogue.

Routes of Administration/Doses Ranitidine may be administered by slow intravenous or intramuscular injection, the dose being 50 mg 6–8-hourly. The oral dose is 150 mg twice daily.

Effects
CVS No effect is seen with normal clinical dosages.
RS The drug has no effect on respiratory parameters.
AS Ranitidine profoundly inhibits gastric acid secretion, reducing the volume, hydrogen ion and pepsin content. The drug has a longer duration of antisecretory activity than cimetidine. Ranitidine has been reported to cause a dose-related increase in lower oesophageal sphincter tone.
Metabolic/Other Ranitidine does not show the antiandrogenic, antidopaminergic or effects on cytochrome P-450 mediated metabolism that are associated with cimetidine. The drug crosses the placenta, but no adverse effects on the fetal well-being have been demonstrated.

Toxicity/Side Effects Reversible abnormalities of liver function tests, rashes and anaphylactoid reactions have been reported following the use of ranitidine. Reversible confusion, thrombocytopenia and leucopenia occur rarely after administration of the drug.

Kinetics

Absorption Ranitidine has an oral bioavailability of 50–60%.

Distribution The drug is approximately 15% protein-bound in the plasma; the V_D is 1.2–1.8 l/kg.

Metabolism A small fraction of the drug is metabolised by oxidation and methylation.

Excretion Ranitidine is predominantly excreted unchanged by the kidney. The clearance is 10 ml/min/kg and the elimination half-life is 1.6–2.5 hours.

Special Points A reduced dosage of the drug should be used in patients with renal failure; the drug is removed by haemodialysis.

Ranitidine may be associated with an increase in nosocomial pneumonia is ventilated critically ill patients.

Remifentanil

Uses   Remifentanil is used to provide the analgesic component of general anaesthesia, and in intensive care.

Chemical   A synthetic anilidopiperidine derivative.

Presentation   As a clear, colourless solution for injection, containing remifentanil hydrochloride in a glycine buffer in 1/2/5 mg vials for dilution prior to infusion.

Main Actions   Analgesia and respiratory depression.

Mode of Action   Remifentanil is a pure mu-agonist; the mu-opioid receptor appears to be specifically involved in the mediation of analgesia. Opioids appear to exert their effects by increasing intracellular calcium concentration which, in turn, increases potassium conductance and hyperpolarisation of excitable cell membranes. The decrease in membrane excitability that results may decrease both pre- and post-synaptic responses.

Route of Administration/Doses   Remifentanil is administered intravenously in boluses of 1 µg/kg and may be infused at a rate of 0.0125–1 µg/kg/min. The peak effect of the drug occurs within 1–3 minutes. The offset is rapid and predictable, even after prolonged infusion.

Effects
CVS   Remifentanil decreases mean arterial pressure and heart rate by 20%. Myocardial contractility and cardiac output may also decrease.
RS   Remifentanil is a potent respiratory depressant, causing a decrease in both the respiratory rate and tidal volume; it also diminishes the ventilatory response to hypoxia and hypercarbia. Chest wall rigidity (the 'wooden chest' phenomenon) may occur after the administration of remifentanil – this may be an effect of the drug on mu-receptors located on GABA-ergic interneurones. The drug does not cause histamine release and thus does not precipitate bronchospasm.
CNS   Remifentanil has a centrally mediated vagal activity. It has an analgesic potency similar to fentanyl and possesses minimal hypnotic or sedative activity. It produces EEG effects similar to those of other opioids – high-amplitude, low-frequency activity. Miosis is produced as a result of stimulation of the Edinger-Westphal nucleus.
AS   The drug decreases gastrointestinal motility; there is a relatively low incidence of nausea and vomiting associated with its use.

Toxicity/Side Effects   Respiratory depression, bradycardia, nausea and vomiting may all complicate the use of remifentanil. Because of its short duration of action, post-operative discomfort may be pronounced if remifentanil is used as a sole analgesic agent peri-operatively.

Kinetics

Distribution Remifentanil has is 70% bound to plasma proteins, two thirds to alpha1-acid protein. The drug has a low lipid solubility compared to other μ opioids, with a low volume of distribution at steady state – $VD_{SS} = 0.25$–0.4 l/kg.

Metabolism Remifentanil undergoes rapid ester hydrolysis by non-specific plasma and tissue esterases to a carboxylic acid derivative, remifentanil acid which is 4,600 fold less potent than remifentanil. The Context Sensitive half-time of remifentanil, 3–5 minutes, does not increase with the duration of infusion unlike other opioids.

Excretion The clearance of remifentanil is 4.2–5 l/min and is independent of renal and hepatic function. The elimination half-life is 5–14 minutes and is unaltered with renal and hepatic dysfunction. The elimination half-life of remifentanil acid is 1.5 hours in healthy individuals but increases to 268 hours with renal failure.

Rocuronium

Uses Rocuronium is used to facilitate intubation and controlled ventilation.

Chemical An aminosteroid which is structurally related to vecuronium.

Presentation As a clear, colourless solution containing 10 mg/ml of rocuronium bromide. The drug is available in 5 and 10 ml ampoules.

Main Action Competitive neuromuscular blockade.

Mode of Action Rocuronium acts by competitive antagonism of acetylcholine at nicotinic (N2) receptors at the post-synaptic membrane of the neuromuscular junction; it also has some pre-junctional action.

Route of Administration/Doses Rocuronium is administered intravenously; the normal intubating dose is 0.6 mg/kg with subsequent doses of one-quarter this amount. The drug may also be infused at a rate of 300–600 µg/kg/hour. Satisfactory intubating conditions are produced within 1 minute – 'priming' does not decrease the onset time of rocuronium. The recovery index is 8–17 minutes. The drug is non-cumulative with repeated administration.

Effects
CVS Rocuronium has minimal cardiovascular effects; with large doses a mild vagolytic effect leads to a slight (9%) increase in heart rate and an increase in mean arterial pressure of up to 16%.
RS Neuromuscular blockade leads to apnoea. Rocuronium does not cause significant histamine release; bronchospasm is extremely uncommon.

Toxicity/Side Effects There have been very rare reports of fatal anaphylactoid reactions with the administration of rocuronium. Cross-sensitivity may exist with vecuronium and pancuronium.

Kinetics

Distribution The drug is 30% protein-bound in the plasma; the V_D is 0.27 l/kg.

Metabolism No metabolites of rocuronium have been detected in plasma or urine.

Excretion Rocuronium is excreted primarily by hepatic uptake and hepatobiliary excretion. 30–40% of the dose is excreted unchanged in the bile; 13–31% in the urine. The clearance is 3.9 ml/kg/min and the elimination half-life is 97 minutes. The pharmacokinetics of rocuronium are not significantly altered in the presence of renal failure. The elimination half-life and duration of action of rocuronium are increased in the presence of hepatic dysfunction.

Special Points The duration of action of rocuronium, in common with other non-depolarising relaxants, may be prolonged by hypokalaemia, hypocalcaemia, hypermagnesaemia, hypoproteinaemia, dehydration, acidosis and hypercapnia. The following drugs, when co-administered with non-depolarising relaxants, increase the effect of the latter: volatile and induction agents, fentanyl, suxamethonium, diuretics, calcium antagonists, alpha- and beta-adrenergic antagonists, protamine, metronidazole and the aminoglycoside antibiotics.

Rocuronium is physically incompatible with thiopentone, methohexitone and diazepam. In animal studies, rocuronium does not appear to be a triggering factor for malignant hyperpyrexia.

Rocuronium causes significantly less rise in intraocular pressure compared to suxamethonium.

Rofecoxib

Uses Rofecoxib is used in the treatment of:
1. osteoarthritis
2. post-operative and dental pain
3. primary dysmenorrhoea and
4. rheumatoid arthritis.

Chemical Furanone.

Presentation As 12.5/25 mg tablets and a suspension containing 2.5/5 mg/ml of rofecoxib.

Main Actions Analgesic, anti-inflammatory and antipyretic.

Mode of Action Rofecoxib is a selective and potent inhibitor of COX-2 enzyme which converts arichidonic acid to cyclic endoperoxides, and thus prevents the formation of prostaglandins and endoperoxides.

Routes of Administration/Doses Rofecoxib is administered orally, in doses of 12.5 mg/day for the treatment of osteoarthritis and up to 50 mg once daily for the management of acute pain.

Toxicity/Side-Effects The drug is generally well tolerated. Insomnia, dizziness, diarrhoea, nausea, headaches and pruritus have been reported. COX-2 inhibitors have a lower incidence of upper gastrointestinal side effects than non-selective NSAIDS.

Effects
GU The drug causes sodium retention and a decrease in the glomerular filtration rate.
Metabolic/Other Naturally occurring pyrexia is reduced by rofecoxib. The drug has no effect on platelet aggregation.

Kinetics

Absorption The drug is well absorbed after oral administration with an oral bioavailability of 93%.

Distribution Rofecoxib is 87% protein-bound in the plasma. The V_D is 1.3 l/kg.

Metabolism The drug is extensively metabolised in the liver, primarily to dihydro derivatives.

Excretion 14% is excreted unchanged in the faeces, 1% unchanged in the urine and the remainder as urinary metabolites. The clearance is 8 l/hr and the elimination half-life is 17 hours.

Special Points Rofecoxib appears to be safe to use in patients with NSAID-induced asthma.

Ropivacaine

Uses Ropivacaine is used as a local anaesthetic.

Chemical An aminoamide which is a member of the pipecoloxylidide group of local anaesthetics.

Presentation As a clear, colourless solution containing 0.2/0.75/1.0% ropivacaine hydrochloride.

Main Action Local anaesthetic.

Mode of Action Local anaesthetics diffuse in their uncharged base form through neural sheaths and the axonal membrane to the internal surface of cell membrane sodium ion channels; here they combine with hydrogen ions to form a cationic species which enters the internal opening of the sodium ion channel and combines with a receptor. This produces blockade of the sodium ion channel, thereby decreasing sodium ion conductance and preventing depolarisation of the cell membrane.

Routes of Administration/Doses Ropivacaine may be administered topically, by infiltration or epidurally; the drug is not currently intended for use in spinal anaesthesia. Sensory blockade is similar in time course to that produced by bupivacaine; motor blockade is slower in onset and shorter in duration than after an equivalent dose of bupivacaine. Alkalinisation of 0.75% ropivacaine significantly increases the duration of epidural blockade.

Effects
CVS Ropivacaine is less cardiotoxic than bupivacaine; in toxic concentrations the drug decreases myocardial contractility, resulting in cardiovascular collapse. Ropivacaine has a biphasic vascular effect causing vasoconstriction at low, but not at high, concentrations.
CNS The principal effect of ropivacaine is reversible neural blockade; this leads to a characteristically biphasic effect in the central nervous system. Initially, excitation (lightheadedness, dizziness, visual and auditory disturbances and fitting) occurs, due to the blockade of inhibitory pathways in the cortex. With increasing doses, depression of both facilitatory and inhibitory pathways occur, leading to central nervous system depression (drowsiness, disorientation and coma). Local anaesthetic agents block neuromuscular transmission when administered intra-arterially; it is thought that a complex of neuro-transmitter, receptor and local anaesthetic is formed which has negligible conductance.
GU Ropivacaine does not compromise uteroplacental circulation.

Toxicity/Side Effects Allergic reactions to the amide-type local anaesthetic agents are extremely rare. The side effects are predominantly correlated with excessive plasma concentrations of the drug, as described above.

Kinetics

Absorption   The absorption of local anaesthetic agents is related to:

1. the site of injection (intercostal > epidural > brachial plexus > subcutaneous)
2. the dose – a linear relationship exists between the total dose and the peak blood concentrations and
3. the presence of vasoconstrictors, which delay absorption.

Distribution   Ropivacaine is 94% protein-bound to alpha-1 acid glycoprotein in the plasma; the V_D is 52–66 l/kg.

Metabolism   Occurs in the liver via cytochrome P-450 to 2,6-pipecoloxylidide.

Excretion   The clearance is 0.82 l/min and the terminal elimination half-life is 59–173 minutes. 86% is excreted in the urine, 1% unchanged.

Special Points   The onset and duration of conduction blockade is related to the pKa, lipid solubility and extent of protein binding of the drug. A low pKa and a high lipid solubility are associated with a rapid onset time; a high degree of protein binding is associated with a long duration of action. The pKa of ropivacaine is 8.1 and the heptane: buffer partition coefficient is 2.9.

Salbutamol

Uses Salbutamol is used in the treatment of:
1. asthma
2. chronic obstructive airways disease and
3. uncomplicated preterm labour.

Chemical A synthetic sympathomimetic amine.

Presentation As 2/4/8 mg tablets, a syrup containing 0.4/2.5 mg/ml, an aerosol delivering 100 µg/puff, a dry powder for inhalation in capsules containing 200/400 µg, a solution for nebulisation containing 2.5/5 mg/ml and as a clear, colourless solution for injection containing 1 mg/ml of salbutamol sulphate.

Main Actions Bronchodilatation and uterine relaxation.

Mode of Action Salbutamol is a beta-adrenergic agonist (with a more pronounced effect at beta-2 than beta-1 receptors) that acts by stimulation of membrane-bound adenyl cyclase in the presence of magnesium ions to increase intracellular cAMP concentrations. It also directly inhibits antigen-induced release of histamine and Slow Releasing Substance of Anaphylaxis from mast cells.

Routes of Administration/Doses The adult oral dose is, 2–4 mg 6–8 hourly. One or two metered puffs of 200–400 µg of the powder may be inhaled 6–8 hourly. 2.5–5 mg of the nebulised solution may similarly be inhaled 6-hourly. The drug may also be administered subcutaneously or intramuscularly in a dose of 0.5 mg 4-hourly. Salbutamol should be administered intravenously as an infusion diluted in dextrose or saline at a rate not exceeding 0.5 µg/kg/min. Bronchodilatation is observed 5–15 minutes after inhalation and 30 minutes after ingestion of the drug and lasts for up to 4 hours.

Effects
CVS In high doses, the beta-1 actions of the drug lead to positive inotropic and chronotropic effect. At lower doses, the beta-2 effects predominate and cause a decrease in the peripheral vascular resistance leading to a decrease in the diastolic blood pressure of 10–20 mmHg.
RS Bronchodilatation, leading to an increased PEFR and FEV_1, occurs after the administration of salbutamol. This is additive to the bronchodilatation produced by phosphodiesterase inhibitors. The drug interferes with the mechanism of hypoxic pulmonary vasoconstriction; an adequate inspired oxygen concentration should be ensured when the drug is used.
GU Salbutamol decreases the tone of the gravid uterus; 10% of an administered dose crosses the placenta and may lead to tachycardia in the fetus.

Metabolic/Other Salbutamol may decrease the plasma potassium concentration by causing a shift of the ion into cells. It may also cause an increase in the plasma concentrations of free fatty acids and glucose; insulin release is therefore stimulated.

Toxicity/Side Effects Anxiety, insomnia, tremor (with no attendant change in motor strength), sweating, palpitations, ketosis, hypokalaemia, postural hypotension and nausea and vomiting may occur following the use of the drug.

Kinetics Data are incomplete.

Absorption 10% of the dose administered by inhalation reaches the bronchial tree, the remainder being swallowed.

Distribution Salbutamol is 8–64% protein-bound in the plasma; the V_D is 156 l.

Metabolism Salbutamol undergoes a significant first-pass metabolism in the liver; the major metabolite is salbutamol 4-O-sulphate.

Excretion 30% of the dose is excreted unchanged in the urine, the remainder in faeces and as the sulphate derivative in the urine. The clearance is 28 l/hour and the elimination half-life is 2.7–5 hours.

Special Points Salbutamol appears to potentiate non-depolarising muscle relaxants.

Sevoflurane

Uses Sevoflurane is used for the induction and maintenance of general anaesthesia.

Chemical A halogenated ether.

Presentation As a clear, colourless liquid which is non-flammable; the commercial preparation contains no additives or stabilisers. The molecular weight of sevoflurane is 200, the boiling point 58.5 °C and the saturated vapour pressure is 21.3 kPa at 20 °C. The MAC of sevoflurane ranges from 1.71 to 2.05 (0.7–2.0 in the presence of 65% nitrous oxide), the oil/gas solubility coefficient is 53 and the blood/gas solubility coefficient 0.6. Sevoflurane is unstable in the presence of moist soda lime, producing small amounts of a sevo-olefin called 'Compound A'. Sevoflurane has a low solubility in rubber and plastics.

Main Action General anaesthesia (reversible loss of both awareness and recall of noxious stimuli).

Mode of Action The mechanism of general anaesthesia remains to be fully elucidated. General anaesthetics appear to disrupt synaptic transmission (especially in the area of the ventrobasal thalamus). The mechanism may include potentiation of gamma-amino-butylic acid and glycine receptors and antagonism at NMDA receptors. Their mode of action at the molecular level appears to involve expansion of hydrophobic regions in the neuronal membrane, either within the lipid phase or within hydrophobic sites in cell membrane proteins.

Route of Administration/Dose Sevoflurane is administered by inhalation; the agent has a pleasant, non-irritant odour. The concentration used for the inhalational induction of anaesthesia is 5–7% and for maintenance 0.5–3%.

Effects

CVS Sevoflurane causes a dose-related decrease in myocardial contractility and mean arterial pressure; systolic pressure decreases to a greater degree than diastolic pressure. The drug has little effect on the heart rate and does not sensitize the myocardium to the effects of catecholamines. Sevoflurane does not appear to cause 'coronary steal'.

RS Sevoflurane causes an increase in respiratory rate; minute volume remains unchanged. The drug depresses the ventilatory response to CO_2 and inhibits hypoxic pulmonary vasoconstriction. Sevoflurane appears to relax bronchial smooth muscle constricted by histamine or acetylcholine.

CNS The principal effect of sevoflurane is general anaesthesia. The drug decreases cerebral vascular resistance and cerebral metabolic rate and increases intracranial pressure in a dose-related manner. Sevoflurane does not cause epileptiform EEG activity.

GU Sevoflurane reduces renal blood flow and leads to a modest increase (comparable to that caused by enflurane) in fluoride ion concentrations. There is no evidence that sevoflurane causes gross changes in human renal function.

Metabolic/Other In animal models the drug decreases liver synthesis of fibrinogen, transferrin and albumin.

Toxicity/Side Effects Sevoflurane acts as a trigger agent for the development of malignant hyperthermia. There are no reports of renal toxicity occurring in patients who have received the drug.

Kinetics

Absorption The major factors affecting the uptake of volatile anaesthetic agents are solubility, cardiac output and the concentration gradient between the alveoli and venous blood. Sevoflurane is exceptionally insoluble in blood; alveolar concentration therefore reaches inspired concentration very rapidly, resulting in a rapid induction of (and emergence from) anaesthesia. An increase in the cardiac output increases the rate of alveolar uptake and slows the induction of anaesthesia. The concentration gradient between alveoli and venous blood approaches zero at equilibrium; a large concentration gradient favours the onset of anaesthesia.

Distribution The drug is initially distributed to organs with a high blood flow (the brain, heart, liver and kidney) and later to less well-perfused organs (muscle, fat and bone).

Metabolism Sevoflurane is metabolised by hepatic cytochrome P-450IIIEI to yield hexafluoroisopropanol, which is further conjugated to its glucuronide. Approximately 3% of the absorbed dose of sevoflurane is metabolised.

Excretion Excretion is via the lungs, predominantly unchanged. Elimination of sevoflurane is rapid due to its low solubility. Peak excretion of hexafluoroisopropanol glucuronide occurs within 12 hours; the elimination half-life is 55 hours.

Special Points Sevoflurane potentiates the action of co-administered depolarising and non-depolarising relaxants to a greater extent than either halothane or enflurane.

Sodium bicarbonate

Uses Sodium bicarbonate is used:
1. for the correction of profound metabolic acidosis, especially that complicating cardiac arrest
2. for the alkalinisation of urine and
3. as an antacid.

Chemical An inorganic salt.

Presentation As 300 mg tablets and as a clear, colourless sterile solution containing 1.26/4.2/8.4% w/v sodium bicarbonate in an aqueous solution. The 8.4% solution contains 1 mmol/ml of sodium and bicarbonate ions and has a calculated osmolarity of 2000 mOsm/l.

Mode of Action The compound freely dissociates to yield bicarbonate ions, which represent the predominant extracellular buffer system. Each gram of sodium bicarbonate will neutralise 12 mEq of hydrogen ions.

Routes of Administration/Doses The adult oral dose for the relief of dyspepsia is 600–1800 mg as required. For the alkalinisation of urine, an oral dose of 3 g is administered every 2 hours until the pH of the urine is >7.

When administered intravenously for the treatment of profound metabolic acidosis, the dose required to restore the pH to normal is usually calculated from the formula:

$$\text{dose (mmol)} = \frac{\text{base deficit (mEq/l)} \times \text{body weight (kg)}}{3}$$

and half this amount administered, before the acid-base status is reassessed.

Effects
CVS Overenthusiastic correction of an acidosis will result in a metabolic alkalosis, which may result in myocardial dysfunction and peripheral tissue hypoxia due to a shift in the oxygen dissociation curve to the left.
RS Metabolic alkalosis diminishes pulmonary ventilation by an effect on the respiratory centre.
CNS The major clinical effect of metabolic alkalosis is excitability of the central nervous system, manifested as nervousness, convulsions, muscle weakness and tetany.
AS Oral administration of the drug results in the release of carbon dioxide with subsequent belching.
Metabolic/Other Hypernatraemia, hyperkalaemia and hypocalcaemia may all result from the intravenous administration of sodium bicarbonate.

Toxicity/Side Effects Hypernatraemia and hyperosmolar syndromes may complicate the use of sodium bicarbonate. The compound is highly irritant to tissues when extravasated and may cause skin necrosis and sloughing.

Kinetics Data are incomplete.

Metabolism Bicarbonate ions react with hydrogen ions to yield carbon dioxide and water.

Excretion Occurs via renal excretion of bicarbonate and exhalation of carbon dioxide.

Special Points Sodium bicarbonate is physically incompatible with calcium salts (which it precipitates) and may cause inactivation of co-administered adrenaline, isoprenaline and suxamethonium.

The use of sodium bicarbonate should be avoided in patients with renal, hepatic or heart failure due to its high sodium content.

Sodium chloride

Uses Sodium chloride is used:
1. to provide maintenance fluid and extracellular fluid replacement
2. to replace sodium and chloride ions under circumstances of reduced intake or excessive loss
3. in the management of hyperosmolar diabetic coma
4. as a priming fluid for haemodialysis and cardiopulmonary bypass machines
5. for rehydration of neonates and infants (0.45% solutions)
6. in the management of severe salt depletion (1.8% solutions)
7. for the dilution of drugs and
8. for interspinous ligament injection in the treatment of chronic neck and back pain (10% solutions).

Chemical An inorganic salt.

Presentation As clear, colourless, sterile 0.45/0.9/1.8/5% solutions in bags of various capacities. The 0.9% solution contains 154 mmol of both sodium and chloride ions per litre. The pH ranges from 4.5–7; they contain no preservative or antimicrobial agents.

Main Action Volume expansion.

Route of Administration/Dose Sodium chloride solutions are administered intravenously at a rate titrated against the patient's clinical status.

Effects
CVS The haemodynamic effects of sodium chloride are proportional to the prevailing circulating volume and are short-lived.
GU Renal perfusion is temporarily restored towards normal in hypovolaemic patients transfused with the crystalloid.

Toxicity/Side Effects The predominant hazard is that of overtransfusion, leading to hypernatraemia or pulmonary oedema.

Kinetics Data are incomplete.

Absorption Sodium chloride is rapidly and completely absorbed when administered orally.

Distribution 0.9% solution is isotonic with extracellular fluid; it is initially distributed into the intravascular compartment where it remains for approximately 30 minutes before being distributed uniformly throughout the extracellular space.

Excretion In the urine.

Sodium nitroprusside

Uses Sodium nitroprusside is used in the management of:
1. hypertensive crises
2. aortic dissection prior to surgery
3. left ventricular failure and
4. to produce hypotension during surgery.

Chemical An inorganic complex.

Presentation As an intravenous solution 10 mg/ml of sodium nitroprusside for dilution prior to infusion it must be protected from light.

Main Actions Vasodilation and hypotension.

Mode of Action Sodium nitroprusside dilates both resistance and capacitance vessels by a direct action on vascular smooth muscle. It appears to act by interacting with sulphydryl groups in the smooth muscle cell membrane, thereby stabilising the membrane and preventing the calcium ion influx necessary for the initiation of contraction.

Route of Administration/Dose Sodium nitroprusside should be administered through a dedicated vein using a controlled infusion device at the rate of 0.5–6 µg/kg/min, titrated according to response. Invasive arterial pressure measurement during the use of the drug is considered mandatory. Onset of action is almost immediate; the desired response is usually achieved in 1–2 minutes.

Effects
CVS In hypertensive and normotensive patients, infusion of the drug causes a decrease in the systemic blood pressure and a compensatory tachycardia; the cardiac output is usually well maintained. In patients with heart failure, cardiac output increases due to a decrease in both venous return and systemic vascular resistance. The myocardial wall tension is decreased and myocardial oxygen consumption falls; the heart rate tends to decrease due to improved haemodynamics with the use of the drug. The blood pressure is usually well maintained under these circumstances. Myocardial contractility is unaltered by the drug.
RS Sodium nitroprusside causes a reversible decrease in P_aO_2 due to attenuation of hypoxic pulmonary vasoconstriction; an increased inspired oxygen concentration may be necessary.
CNS The drug causes cerebral vasodilation, leading to an increase in intracranial pressure in normocapnic patients; a 'steal' phenomenon may occur. The autoregulatory curve is shifted to the left.
AS Sodium nitroprusside decreases to lower oesophageal sphincter pressure and may cause a paralytic ileus.

GU   The renal blood flow and glomerular filtration rate are well maintained during infusions of the drug.

Metabolic/Other   A compensatory increase in plasma cate-cholamine concentration and plasma renin activity occur during the use of the drug. A metabolic acidosis may also occur.

Toxicity/Side Effects   The major disadvantage of the drug is its liability to produce cyanide toxicity, the likelihood of which is increased by hypothermia, malnutrition, vitamin B_{12} deficiency and severe renal or hepatic impairment. Cyanide ion toxicity is related to the rate of infusion of sodium nitroprusside rather than to the total dose used; however, it is recommended that no more than 1.5 mg/kg of the drug is infused acutely, and no more than 4 μg/kg/min is used chronically. The cyanide ion combines with cytochrome C and leads to impairment of aerobic metabolism; metabolic acidosis due to an increased serum lactic acid concentration may result. The signs of cyanide ion toxicity are tachycardia, dysrhythmias, hyperventilation, sweating and the development of a metabolic acidosis; these occur at plasma cyanide ion concentrations in excess of 8 μg/ml. Treatment of cyanide ion toxicity involves curtailing the infusion of sodium nitroprusside, general supportive measures and the administration of sodium thiosulphate or dicobalt edetate.

Additionally, profound hypotension produced by the drug may manifest itself as nausea and vomiting, abdominal pain, restlessness, headache, dizziness, palpitations and retrosternal pain.

Kinetics   Pharmacokinetic data are difficult to obtain, due to the very short duration of action of the drug.

Absorption   The drug is not absorbed orally.

Distribution   Sodium nitroprusside in the blood is confined essentially to the plasma; scarcely any is present within red blood cells. The V_D is approximately the same as the extracellular space (15 l).

Metabolism   Occurs by two separate pathways: in the presence of low plasma concentrations of sodium nitroprusside, the predominant route appears to be by reaction with the sulphydryl groups of amino acids present in the plasma. In the presence of higher plasma concentrations of the drug, rapid non-enzymatic hydrolysis occurs within red blood cells. Five cyanide ions are produced by the degradation of each molecule of sodium nitroprusside; one reacts with methaemoglobin to form cyanomethaemoglobin. The remaining four cyanide ions enter the plasma; 80% of these react with thiosulphate in a reaction catalysed by hepatic rhodanese to form thiocyanate. The remainder of the cyanide ions react with hydroxy-cobalamin to form cyanocobalamin (vitamin B_{12}).

Sodium nitroprusside

Excretion Both thiocyanate and cyanocobalamin are excreted unchanged in the urine. The elimination half-life of the former is 2.7 days.

Special Points Sodium nitroprusside is removed by haemodialysis.

Sodium valproate

Uses   Sodium valproate is used in the treatment of:
1. primary generalised epilepsies, especially petit mal epilepsy, myoclonic seizures, infantile spasms and tonic-clonic epilepsy
2. chronic pain of non-malignant origin.

Chemical   Sodium valproate is the sodium salt of valproic acid, a fatty (carboxylic) acid.

Presentation   As 100/200/500 mg tablets, a syrup containing 40 mg/ml and in ampoules containing 400 mg of lyophilised soium valproate for dilution in 4 ml of water.

Main Action   Anticonvulsant.

Mode of Action   The most likely mode of action is via GABA-ergic inhibition; sodium valproate increases brain GABA levels by inhibition of succinic semialdehyde dehydrogenase in the GABA shunt. Alternatively it may:
1. mimic the action of GABA at post-synaptic receptors and
2. reduce excitatory inhibition (especially that due to aspartate).

Routes of Administration/Doses   The adult oral dose is 600–2500 mg daily in two divided doses. The intravenous dose is 400–2500 mg daily in divided doses. The effective plasma range is 40–100 mg/l.

Effects
CNS   The drug has anticonvulsant properties as described. Sodium valproate produces minimal sedation; an essential tremor may occasionally develop with the use of the drug.
Metabolic/Other   Hyperammonaemia occurs infrequently.

Toxicity/Side Effects   Sodium valproate is generally well tolerated. Hepatic dysfunction, acute pancreatitis, gastrointestinal upsets, hair loss, oedema and weight gain may occur following administration of the drug. There are also reports of platelet disturbances (decreased platelet aggregation and thrombocytopenia) and coagulation disturbances (increased bleeding time, prothrombin time and partial activated thromboplastin time) complicating the administration of sodium valproate.

Kinetics

Absorption   Sodium valproate is rapidly and completely absorbed; the oral bioavailability is virtually 100%.

Distribution   The drug is 90% protein-bound in the plasma, predominantly to albumin; the V_D is 0.1–0.41 l/kg. Brain concentrations are 7–28% of plasma levels.

154

Metabolism Sodium valproate is almost completely metabolised in the liver by oxidation and glucuronidation; some of the metabolites are active.

Excretion 1–3% is excreted unchanged in the urine. The clearance is 7–11 ml/kg/hour and the elimination half-life is 8–20 hours.

Special Points High concentrations of sodium valproate displace thiopentone from its binding sites *in vitro* and similarly displace diazepam *in vivo*. Platelet function may need to be monitored prior to surgery or epidural or spinal anaesthesia.

The drug is contraindicated in patients with acute liver disease, and liver function should be monitored during chronic therapy. The sedative effects of the drug are additive with those of other central nervous system depressants.

Sodium valproate is not removed by dialysis.

Spironolactone

Uses   Spironolactone is used in the treatment of:
1. congestive cardiac failure
2. hepatic cirrhosis with ascites and oedema
3. refractory oedema
4. hypertension
5. the nephrotic syndrome
6. in combination with loop or thiazide diuretics to conserve potassium and
7. in the diagnosis and treatment of Conn's syndrome.

Chemical   A synthetic steroid.

Presentation   As 25/50/100 mg tablets of spironolactone. Fixed-dose combinations with hydroflumethiazide or frusemide are also available.

Main Action   Diuretic.

Mode of Action   Spironolactone acts as a competitive antagonist of aldosterone at the latter's receptor site in the distal convoluted tubule; consequently, sodium ion reabsorption is inhibited and potassium ion reabsorption is increased. The drug thus promotes saliuresis and also potentiates that produced by other diuretic agents.

Routes of Administration/Doses   The adult oral dose of spironolactone is 100–400 mg daily; the corresponding dose of potassium canrenoate is 200–800 mg administered by slow intravenous infusion. The drug has a slow onset of action; the diuretic effect takes 3 to 4 days to become established.

Effects
CVS   The drug has an antihypertensive effect that may be mediated by alteration of the extracellular:intracellular sodium ion gradient or by antagonism of the effect of aldosterone on arteriolar smooth muscle.
CNS   Spironolactone may produce both sedation and muscular weakness, presumably secondarily to electrolyte derangements.
GU   The principal effect of the drug is diuresis, with retention of potassium ions. The renal blood flow and glomerular filtration rate are unaffected although the free water clearance may increase.
Metabolic/Other   Spironolactone has an antiandrogenic effect, due to inhibition of ovarian androgen secretion and interference with the peripheral action of endogenous androgens. The drug increases renal calcium ion excretion, and may also lead to a reversible hyperchloraemic metabolic acidosis and an increased plasma urea concentration.

Toxicity/Side Effects The predominant side effect of spironolactone is hyperkalaemia, especially in the presence of renal impairment. The use of the drug is also associated with an appreciable incidence of nausea and vomiting and other gastrointestinal disturbances. Menstrual irregularities in the female and gynaecomastia in the male may result from the antiandrogenic effects of spironolactone.

Kinetics

Absorption Spironolactone is incompletely absorbed when administered orally and has a bioavailability by this route of 70%; the drug undergoes extensive first-pass hepatic metabolism.

Distribution The drug is >90% protein-bound in the plasma.

Metabolism Spironolactone is rapidly and extensively metabolised by deacetylation and dethiolation; some of the metabolites, including canrenone, are active.

Excretion The metabolites are principally excreted in the urine, with a small proportion undergoing biliary excretion. The elimination half-life of spironolactone is 1–2 hours.

Special Points Spironolactone decreases the responsiveness to co-administered pressor agents and increases the effects of co-administered cardiovascular depressants, including anaesthetic agents. The drug increases the serum concentrations of co-administered digoxin and may interfere with digoxin assay techniques.

Streptokinase

Uses Streptokinase is used:
1. in the treatment of acute myocardial infarction
2. for the intravascular dissolution of thrombi and emboli, e.g. deep vein thrombosis and pulmonary embolus and
3. in the treatment of acute or subacute occlusion of peripheral arteries.

Chemical A protein obtained from Group C beta-haemolytic streptococci.

Presentation As a freeze-dried powder in vials containing 250 000/750 000/1.5 million units of streptokinase.

Main Actions Fibrinolysis.

Mode of Action Streptokinase acts indirectly on plasmin; the first phase is the formation of a streptokinase–plasminogen activator complex which then converts further plasminogen molecules to active plasmin. Plasmin then digests fibrin to produce lysis of thrombi.

Routes of Administration/Doses Streptokinase is infused intravenously (either peripherally or centrally at the site of occlusion) in 50–200 ml of saline, dextrose or gelatin. For the treatment of acute myocardial infarction, 1.5 million units are infused over a period of 1 hour. For the dissolution of thrombi or emboli, 250 000 units are infused over 30 minutes; subsequently, 100 000 units are infused per hour for 24–72 hours. Therapy should be monitored by either the thrombin time (which should be 2–5 times the control value) or prothrombin time.

Effects
CVS Transient hypotension and dysrhythmias may occur following the administration of streptokinase.
Metabolic/Other Fibrinolysis is produced by the action of the drug on plasmin.

Toxicity/Side Effects Excessive haemorrhage may complicate the use of the drug; if serious, this should be treated by cessation of Streptokinase therapy, resuscitation and intravenous tranexamic acid (10 mg/kg). Pyrexia occurs commonly. Allergic reactions may occur, particularly on repeated exposure, as streptokinase is markedly antigenic. This can be minimised by steroid and antihistamine pretreatment. Poly-neuropathy has occasionally been reported following the use of the drug.

Kinetics Data are incomplete.

Excretion The elimination half-life is 83 minutes.

Special Points   Clotting factors return to normal values 24 hours after cessation of therapy; this is the time interval advisable before invasive procedures are undertaken.

Treatment with anticoagulants (including dextrans) or any drug which affects platelet function or formation increases the danger of haemorrhage.

Heparinisation may be indicated to prevent further thrombosis after initial treatment with streptokinase.

Sucralfate

Uses Sucralfate is used:
1. in the treatment of peptic ulcer disease and
2. for the prevention of stress ulceration in the critically ill.

Chemical An aluminium salt of sulphated sucrose.

Presentation As tablets containing 1 g sucralfate and a white, viscous suspension containing 200 mg/ml of sucralfate.

Main Actions Cytoprotection of the upper gastrointestinal tract.

Mode of Action At acid pH sucralfate forms a viscous paste which adheres preferentially to peptic ulcers via ionic binding. It acts by providing a physical barrier to the diffusion of acid, pepsin and bile salts and also by forming complexes with proteins at the ulcer surface which resist peptic hydrolysis.

Routes of Administration/Doses The adult dose for the prophylaxis of stress ulceration is 1 g 6-hourly.

Effects
AS Sucralfate has weak intrinsic antacid activity. It has no effect on gastric emptying time. The drug increases gastric blood flow and enhances gastric epithelial proliferation via stimulation of gastric mucosal epidermal growth factor and fibroblast growth factor.
Metabolic/Other In uraemic patients sucralfate increases aluminium absorption and therefore should be used with care. It acts as a phosphate binder which may induce hypophosphataemia.

Toxicity/Side Effects Sucralfate is essentially non-toxic. Constipation occurs in 2%.

Kinetics

Absorption Sucralfate is minimally (3–5%) absorbed after oral administration.

Distribution 85–95% of an oral dose remains in the gastrointestinal tract. The V_D and percentage protein binding are unknown.

Metabolism No metabolism of the drug occurs in man.

Excretion Predominantly unchanged in the faeces. The fraction that is absorbed is excreted primarily in the urine.

Sufentanil

Uses   Sufentanil is used for:
1. the induction and maintenance of general anaesthesia and has been used for
2. post-operative analgesia.

Chemical   A phenylpiperidine which is the thienyl derivative of fentanyl.

Presentation   As a clear solution containing 50 µg/ml of sufentanil citrate. The drug is not commercially available in the United Kingdom.

Main Action   Analgesia and respiratory depression.

Mode of Action   Sufentanil is a highly selective mu-agonist; the mu-opioid receptor appears to be specifically involved in the mediation of analgesia. Part of the analgesic effect of the drug may be attributable to stimulation of 5-HT release. Opioids appear to exert their effects by increasing intracellular calcium concentration which, in turn, increases potassium conductance and hyperpolarisation of excitable cell membranes. The decrease in membrane excitability that results may decrease both pre- and post-synaptic responses.

Routes of Administration/Doses   The intravenous dose is 0.5–50 µg/kg and the adult dose via the epidural route is 10–100 µg (the optimal post-operative dose being 30–50 µg. When administered intravenously, the drug acts in 1–6 minutes and the duration of effect is 0.5–8 hours, dependent on the other components of the anaesthetic.

Effects
CVS   Sufentanil causes little haemodynamic disturbance. Heart rate and blood pressure tend to decrease immediately post-induction. Venous pooling may lead to orthostatic hypotension.
RS   The drug produces dose-dependent respiratory depression, which may be delayed in onset. Chest wall rigidity (the 'wooden chest' phenomenon) may occur after the administration of sufentanil – this may be an effect of the drug on mu-receptors located on GABA-ergic interneurones.
CNS   Sufentanil is 2000–4000 times as potent an analgesic as morphine. The EEG changes produced by the drug are similar to those produced by fentanyl: initial beta activity is decreased and alpha activity is increased; subsequently alpha activity disappears and delta activity predominates. The drug has no intrinsic effect on intracranial pressure. Miosis is produced as a result of stimulation of the Edinger-Westphal nucleus.
AS   Sufentanil appears to cause less nausea than fentanyl. The drug may cause spasm of the sphincter of Oddi.

162

Metabolic/Other The drug tends to obtund the stress response to surgery, although it does not completely abolish it. Sufentanil may cause histamine release and may have less effect on immune function than fentanyl.

Toxicity/Side Effects Hypotension, tachycardia, bradycardia, nausea and the 'wooden chest' phenomenon are the side effects most commonly reported with the use of sufentanil. Tonic/clonic movements of the limbs have also been reported.

Kinetics

Absorption The drug is normally administered intravenously; the drug is, however, 20% absorbed when administered transdermally.

Distribution Sufentanil is 92% protein-bound in the plasma, predominantly to alpha-1 acid glycoprotein. The drug is highly lipophilic; the V_D is 1.74–5.17 l/kg.

Metabolism The metabolic pathways are unknown in man, although two metabolites (norsufentanil and desmethyl-sufentanil) have been identified in the urine.

Excretion 60% of an administered dose appear in the urine and 10% in bile. The clearance is 11–21 ml/min/kg; the elimination half-life is 119–175 minutes.

Special Points Sufentanil decreases the MAC of co-administered volatile agents by 60–70%. The drug should be used with caution in the presence of renal or hepatic failure although the kinetics appear to be unaltered.

The drug increases the effect of non-depolarising muscle relaxants to a similar extent to halothane.

Suxamethonium

Uses Suxamethonium is used:
1. wherever rapid and profound neuromuscular blockade is required, e.g. to facilitate tracheal intubation and
2. for the modification of fits after electroconvulsive therapy.

Chemical The dicholine ester of succinic acid (equivalent to two acetylcholine molecules joined back-to-back).

Presentation As a clear aqueous solution containing 50 mg/ml of suxamethonium chloride – the preparation should be stored at 4 °C.

Main Actions Neuromuscular blockade of brief duration in skeletal muscle.

Mode of Action Suxamethonium causes prolonged depolarisation of skeletal muscle fibres to a membrane potential above which an action potential can be triggered.

Routes of Administration/Doses The intravenous dose is 0.5–2.0 mg/kg; the onset of action occurs within 30 seconds and the duration of action is 3–5 minutes. Infusion of a 0.1% solution at 2–15 mg/kg/hr will yield 90% twitch depression. The intramuscular dose is up to 2.5 mg/kg. Equal doses on a mg/kg basis have a shorter duration of action in infants.

Effects
CVS With repeated doses of suxamethonium, bradycardia and a slight increase in mean arterial pressure may occur.
RS Apnoea occurs subsequent to skeletal muscle paralysis.
CNS The administration of suxamethonium may initially cause fasciculations which are then followed by a phase I depolarising block. The characteristics of this during partial paralysis are:
1. a well-sustained tetanus during stimulation at 50–100 Hz
2. the absence of post-tetanic facilitation
3. a train-of-four ratio of greater than 0.7 and
4. potentiation by anticholinesterases.

With repeated administration or a large total dose a phase II block may develop. The characteristics of this during partial paralysis are:
1. a poorly sustained tetanus
2. post-tetanic facilitation
3. a train-of-four ratio of less than 0.3
4. reversal by anticholinesterases and
5. tachyphylaxis.

Intracranial and intraocular pressure are both raised following the administration of suxamethonium.
AS The intragastric pressure increases by 7–12 cmH$_2$O; the lower oesophageal sphincter tone simultaneously decreases

with the use of suxamethonium. Salivation and gastric secretion are increased.

Metabolic/Other Serum potassium concentration is briefly increased in normal individuals by 0.2–0.4 mmol/l.

Toxicity/Side Effects Bradycardia and other dysrhythmias may occur with single or repeated dosing. The hyperkalaemic response is markedly exaggerated in patients with burns or major denervation of muscle and acute or chronic renal failure; this may lead to cardiac arrest. Postoperative muscular pains are common, especially in women, the middleaged and those ambulant early in the post-operative period. Intraocular pressure is transiently raised following the use of suxamethonium—the drug should be used with caution in patients with penetrating eye injuries. Suxamethonium is a potent trigger agent for the development of malignant hyper-thermia, and may cause generalised contractures in those patients exhibiting myotonia. Prolonged apnoea may occur in susceptible individuals (*v.i.*). There have been many reports of fatal anaphylactoid reactions with the administration of Suxamethonium. Cross sensitivity exists with many of the non depolarising drugs following administration of Suxamethonium.

Kinetics

Distribution An initial rapid redistribution phase may contribute to the brief duration of action of the drug. Suxamethonium appears to be protein-bound to an unknown extent.

Metabolism The drug is hydrolysed by plasma cholinesterase (EC 3.1.1.8) to succinylomonocholine (which is weakly active) and choline; the former is further hydrolysed by plasma cholinesterase to succinic acid and choline. 80% of an administered dose is hydrolysed before it reaches the neuromuscular junction.

Excretion 2–10% of an administered dose is excreted unchanged in the urine. The *in vivo* hydrolysis rate is 3–7 mg/l/min and the half-life 2.7–4.6 minutes.

Special Points The incidence of muscle pains after the administration of suxamethonium may be decreased by pretreatment with:
1. a low (0.2 mg/kg) dose of suxamethonium
2. a small dose of a non-depolarising relaxant
3. diazepam
4. dantrolene
5. aspirin or
6. vitamin C.

Plasma cholinesterase activity may be influenced by both genetic and acquired factors, leading to an altered pattern of response to suxamethonium. The normal gene encoding for plasma cholinesterase is E_I^u (usual); three abnormal genes also exist: E_I^a (atypical), E_I^s (silent) and E_I^f (fluoride-resistant).

Simple Mendelian genetics are involved; 94% of the population are heterozygous for the usual gene and are clinically normal in their response to suxamethonium. E_I^a homozygotes comprise 0.03%, E_I^s homozygotes 0.001% and E_I^f homozygotes 0.0003% of the population and all remain apnoeic for 1–2 hours after receiving the drug and develop a phase II block during this period (fresh frozen plasma may be used to provide a source of plasma cholinesterase under these circumstances). All possible combinations of heterozygote exist – they constitute 3.8% of the population and remain apnoeic for approximately 10 minutes after receiving suxamethonium.

In addition, plasma cholinesterase concentrations may be reduced in pregnancy, liver disease, cardiac or renal failure, hypoproteinaemic states, carcinomatosis, thyrotoxicosis, tetanus, muscular dystrophy and in patients with burns, and suxamethonium may have a prolonged action in these states. Drugs which decrease the activity of plasma cholinesterase include ecothiopate, tacrine, procaine, lignocaine, lithium and magnesium salts, ketamine, pancuronium, the oral contraceptive pill, and cytotoxic agents. Suxamethonium does not appear to be potentiated by volatile agents, although phase II block may appear more readily in their presence.

Suxamethonium is pharmaceutically incompatible with thiopentone. The effects of digoxin may be enhanced by suxamethonium, leading to enhanced ventricular excitability.

Temazepam

Uses Temazepam is used:
1. as a hypnotic and
2. for anaesthetic premedication.

Chemical A 3-hydroxy benzodiazepine which is a minor metabolite of diazepam.

Presentation As capsules containing 10/15/20/30 mg, and an elixir containing 2 mg/ml of temazepam.

Main Actions Temazepam has anxiolytic, hypnotic, anticonvulsant and muscle-relaxant properties.

Mode of Action Benzodiazepines are thought to act via specific benzodiazepine receptors found at synapses throughout the central nervous system, but concentrated especially in the cortex and mid-brain. Benzodiazepine receptors are closely linked with GABA receptors, and appear to facilitate the activity of the latter. Activated GABA receptors open chloride ion channels which then either hyperpolarise or short-circuit the synaptic membrane.

Route of Administration/Dose Temazepam is administered orally; the adult dose is 10–60 mg.

Effects
CVS Benzodiazepines have minimal effects on cardiovascular parameters; an insignificant decrease in blood pressure may occur. Benzodiazepines can dilate coronary blood vessels whilst simultaneously reducing myocardial oxygen consumption.
RS High doses (>40 mg) decrease the ventilatory response to hypercapnia.
CNS The drug causes muscular relaxation, sedation, hypnosis and axiolysis; it also has anticonvulsant properties.
Metabolic/Other High (>40 mg) doses cause a slight fall in temperature.

Toxicity/Side Effects Temazepam is normally well tolerated; gastrointestinal upsets, headaches, dreams, paraesthesiae and a 'hangover effect' (in 10–15%) may occur. Tolerance and dependence may occur with prolonged use of benzodiazepines; acute withdrawal of benzodiazepines in these circumstances may produce insomnia, anxiety, confusion, psychosis and perceptual disturbances.

Kinetics

Absorption Absorption of oral temazepam is virtually complete; antacids delay the absorption of benzodiazepines.

Distribution Temazepam is 76% protein-bound *in vitro*. The V_D is 0.8 l/kg.

Metabolism   The drug is predominantly metabolised in the liver by direct conjugation to glucuronide; active metabolites are not formed to any great extent.

Excretion   80% of an administered dose appears in the urine as inactive conjugates; 12% is excreted in the faeces. The clearance is 6.6 l/hour and the elimination half-life is 5–11 hours.

Special Points   The drug is not removed by haemodialysis. Temazepam is a drug of abuse and has controlled drug status.

Terbutaline

Uses   Terbutaline is used in the treatment of:
1. asthma
2. chronic obstructive airways disease and
3. uncomplicated preterm labour.

Chemical   An alcohol.

Presentation   As 5/7.5 mg tablets, a syrup containing 0.3 mg/ml, a clear solution for injection containing 0.5 mg/ml, a respirator solution containing 2.5/10 mg/ml and as an inhaler delivering 0.25/0.5 μg per actuation of terbutaline sulphate. It can be administered intravenously 250–500 μg 6-hourly, and by infusion at a rate up to 5 μg/min per adults.

Main Actions   Bronchodilatation and uterine relaxation.

Mode of Action   Terbutaline is a beta-adrenergic agonist (with a more pronounced effect at beta-2 than beta-1 receptors) that acts by stimulation of membrane-bound adenyl cyclase in the presence of magnesium ions to increase intracellular cAMP concentrations.

Routes of Administration/Doses   The adult oral dose is 2.5–5 mg 8-hourly; the subcutaneous, intramuscular and intravenous dose is 0.25–0.5 mg once or twice a day. Terbutaline may be administered by intravenous infusion diluted in dextrose or saline at the rate of 1.5–5 μg/min for 8–10 hours. The dose by inhalation is 0.25–0.5 μg 4-hourly or 2–5 mg 8–12-hourly if nebulised.

Effects
CVS   When used in large doses, terbutaline has positive inotropic and chronotropic effects.
RS   Bronchodilatation, leading to an increased PEFR and FEV_1, occurs after administration of the drug. This is additive to the bronchodilatation produced by phosphodiesterase inhibitors. The drug interferes with the mechanism of hypoxic pulmonary vasoconstriction; an adequate inspired oxygen concentration should be ensured when terbutaline is used.
GU   Terbutaline relaxes uterine musculature. An increased tendency to bleeding has been reported in association with Caesarean section.
Metabolic/Other   Hyperinsulinaemia, leading to hypoglycaemia and hypokalaemia, may follow administration of the drug. Antepartum administration of terbutaline stimulates release of surface-active material into the alveolar space of the fetus, improving the function of the neonatal lung.

Toxicity/Side Effects   Tremor, palpitations, cramps, anxiety and headache occur uncommonly after the administration of terbutaline.

Kinetics

Absorption The drug is incompletely absorbed after oral administration; the bioavailability is 7–26%. Less than 10% is absorbed after inhalation, the remainder being swallowed.

Distribution Terbutaline is 25% protein-bound in the plasma; the V_D is 1.6 l/kg.

Metabolism Terbutaline has an extensive first-pass metabolism; the drug is predominantly metabolised to a sulphate conjugate.

Excretion 60–70% is excreted unchanged in the urine; the remainder as the sulphated conjugate. The clearance is 1.75–2.75 ml/min/kg and the elimination half-life is 11.5–23 hours.

Tetracycline

Uses   Tetracycline is used in the treatment of infections of:
1. the respiratory, gastrointestinal and urinary tracts
2. ear, nose and throat
3. soft tissues and in the treatment of
4. venereal diseases, including non-specific urethritis
5. typhus fever
6. psittacosis
7. cholera
8. acne rosacea and for
9. the treatment of recurrent pleural effusions and
10. the prophylaxis of subacute bacterial endocarditis.

Chemical   A napthacenecarboxamide derivative.

Presentation   As 250 mg tablets, a syrup containing 25 mg/ml, in vials containing 100 mg (with procaine) for intramuscular injection and 250/500 mg (with ascorbic acid) for intravenous injection of tetracycline hydrochloride. An ointment for topical use is also available.

Main Actions   Tetracycline is a broad spectrum bacteriostatic antibiotic which is active against Gram-positive and Gram-negative bacteria, including *Clostridium*, *Streptococcus*, *Neisseria*, *Brucella* and *Vibrio* sp., *Haemophilus influenzae*, *Yersinia pestis* and rickettsiae, *Mycoplasma*, *Chlamydia*, *Leptospira* and *Treponema* sp.

Mode of Action   Tetracycline inhibits bacterial protein synthesis by binding to bacterial 30S ribosomes (in the same manner as do aminoglycosides) and preventing the access of aminoacyl tRNA to the mRNA-ribosome complex, thereby preventing further elongation of the polypeptide chain.

Routes of Administration/Doses   The adult oral dose is 250–500 mg 6-hourly. The corresponding intramuscular dose is 100 mg 4–8-hourly and the intravenous dose is 0.5–1 g 12-hourly. The intrapleural dose is 500 mg (of the intravenous preparation). Intramuscular injection of the drug is painful.

Effects
CVS   Tetracycline may increase intracranial pressure.
Metabolic/Other   The drug may cause an increase in the plasma urea concentration and decrease the plasma prothrombin activity.

Toxicity/Side Effects   Occur in 1–5% of patients. The drug may cause renal and hepatic impairment, gastrointestinal and haematological disturbances, moniliasis, rashes, photosensitivity and thrombophlebitis. Tetracycline may also cause tooth staining in infancy.

Kinetics

Absorption Tetracycline is incompletely absorbed when administered orally (it chelates with iron, calcium and aluminium in the gut). The bioavailability is 77% by the oral route.

Distribution The drug is widely distributed and exhibits good tissue penetration. The drug is 62–68% protein-bound in the plasma; the V_D is 0.75–1.37 l/kg.

Metabolism 5% of the dose is metabolised to epitetracycline, the remainder is excreted unchanged.

Excretion 95% of the dose is excreted unchanged; 60% is excreted in the urine by glomerular filtration, the remainder in the faeces. The clearance is 1.43–1.91 ml/min/kg and the half-life is 10–16 hours. A decreased dose should be used in the presence of renal failure.

Special Points Tetracycline has been demonstrated to increase the action of non-depolarising relaxants. It is pharmaceutically incompatible with a host of other drugs, including thiopentone, sodium bicarbonate and autologous blood.

Thiopentone

Uses Thiopentone is used:
1. for the induction of anaesthesia
2. in the management of status epilepticus and has been used
3. for brain protection.

Chemical A thiobarbiturate.

Presentation As a hygroscopic yellow powder, containing thiopentone sodium and 6% sodium carbonate stored under an atmosphere of nitrogen. The drug is reconstituted in water prior to use to yield a 2.5% solution with a pH of 10.8 and pKa of 7.6 which is stable in solution for 24–48 hours.

Main Actions Hypnotic and anticonvulsant.

Mode of Action Barbiturates are thought to act primarily at synapses by depressing post-synaptic sensitivity to neurotransmitters and by impairing pre-synaptic neurotransmitter release. Multi-synaptic pathways are depressed preferentially; the reticular activating system is particularly sensitive to the depressant effects of barbiturates. The action of barbiturates at the molecular level is unknown. They may act in a manner analogous to that of local anaesthetic agents by entering cell membranes in the unionised form, subsequently becoming ionised and exerting a membrane-stabilising effect by decreasing sodium and potassium ion conductance, decreasing the amplitude of the action potential and slowing the rate of conduction in excitable tissue. In high concentrations, barbiturates depress the enzymes involved in glucose oxidation, inhibit the formation of ATP and depress calcium-dependent action potentials. They also inhibit calcium-dependent neurotransmitter release and enhance chloride ion conductance in the absence of GABA.

Routes of Administration/Doses The dose by the intravenous route is 2–7 mg/kg; following bolus administration, thiopentone acts in one arm–brain circulation time and lasts for 5–15 minutes; it is cumulative with repeated administration. The drug may also be administered rectally in a dose of 1 g/22 kg body weight, when it acts within 15 minutes.

Effects
CVS Thiopentone is a negative inotrope and decreases cardiac output by approximately 20%; the blood pressure usually decreases as a result of both this effect and a decrease in systemic vascular resistance.

RS Thiopentone is a potent respiratory depressant; following intravenous administration a period of apnoea may occur, followed by a more prolonged period of respiratory depression with a decrease in ths ventilatory response to hypercapnia.

Laryngeal spasm is occasionally seen in association with the administration of thiopentone; the drug may also produce a degree of bronchoconstriction.

CNS Thiopentone produces a smooth, rapid induction of anaesthesia. Cerebral blood flow, intracranial pressure and intraocular pressure are all decreased after the administration of the drug. As with all barbiturates, thiopentone has anticonvulsant properties. The drug is antanalgesic when used in small doses. The characteristic EEG changes observed after thiopentone administration are initially a fast activity which is subsequently replaced by synchronised low-frequency waves.

AS The drug causes some depression of intestinal activity and constriction of the splanchnic vasculature.

GU Thiopentone decreases renal plasma flow and increases ADH secretion, leading to a decrease in urine output. It has no effect on the tone of the gravid uterus.

Metabolic/Other A slight transient decrease in the serum potassium concentration may occur following the administration of thiopentone.

Toxicity/Side Effects Severe anaphylactoid reactions may occur with the use of the drug, with a reported incidence of 1 in 20 000. Extravasation of the drug may lead to tissue necrosis; inadvertent intra-arterial injection may lead to arterial constriction and thrombosis. The treatment of the latter includes the administration of analgesia and alpha-adrenergic antagonists, sympathetic blockade of the limb and anticoagulation.

Kinetics

Absorption Thiopentone is absorbed when administered orally or rectally.

Distribution The drug is 65–86% protein-bound in the plasma, predominantly to albumin; 40% is sequestered in red blood cells; the V_D is 1.96 l/kg. The rapid onset of action of the drug is due to:
1. the high blood flow to the brain
2. the lipophilicity of the drug and
3. its low degree of ionisation – only the non-ionised fraction crosses the blood–brain barrier (thiopentone is 61% non-ionised at pH 7.4: hyperventilation increases the non-bound fraction and increases the anaesthetic effect).

The relatively brief duration of anaesthesia following a bolus of thiopentone is due to redistribution to muscle and later to fat.

Metabolism Occurs in the liver by side-arm oxidation, oxidation to pentobarbitone and ring cleavage to form urea and 3-carbon fragments. 15% of the dose of the drug is metabolised per hour; 30% may remain in the body 24 hours after administration.

Thiopentone

Excretion Occurs predominantly in the urine as inactive metabolites; 0.5% is excreted unchanged. The clearance is 2.7–4.1 ml/kg/min and the elimination half life is 3.4–22 hours.

Special Points Volatile agents and surgery have no effect on the V_D or clearance of thiopentone; morphine increases the hypnotic effect of the drug and increases its brain half-life. The drug may induce acute clinical and biochemical manifestations in patients with porphyria. Thiopentone should be used with caution in patients with fixed cardiac output states, hepatic or renal dysfunction, myxoedema, dystrophia myotonica, myasthenia gravis, familial periodic paralysis, and in the elderly or in patients who are hypovolaemic.

Thiopentone is not removed by dialysis.

Thyroxine/ Triiodothyronine

Uses   Thyroid hormones are used in the treatment of:
1.   hypothyroidism
2.   myxoedema coma and
3.   goitre.

Chemical   Both hormones are iodine-containing amino acid derivatives of thyronine.

Presentation   Thyroxine is presented as tablets containing $50/100\,\mu g$ of thyroxine sodium. Triiodothyronine is presented as $20\,\mu g$ tablets and a white lyophilised powder for reconstitution in water containing $20\,\mu g$ of triiodothyronine.

Main Actions   Modulation of growth and metabolism.

Mode of Action   The thyroid hormones, probably predominantly triiodothyronine, combine with a 'receptor protein' within the cell nucleus and thereby activate the DNA transcription process leading to an increase in the rate of RNA synthesis and a generalised increase in protein synthesis.

Routes of Administration/Doses   The adult oral dose of thyroxine is $25–300\,\mu g$ daily in divided doses, titrated according to the clinical response and results of thyroid function tests. The corresponding dose of triiodothyronine is $10–60\,\mu g$ daily; the dose by the intravenous route is $5–20\,\mu g$ 4–12 hourly; close monitoring is essential during intravenous administration. There is a 24 hour latency period before the effects of thyroxine are manifested; the peak effect occurs in 6–7 days. Triiodothyronine acts in 6 hours and the peak effect is observed within 24 hours.

Effects
CVS   The thyroid hormones are positively inotropic and chronotropic; these effects may be mediated by an increase in the number of myocardial beta-adrenergic receptors. The systolic blood pressure is increased by $10–20\,mmHg$; the diastolic blood pressure decreases and mean arterial pressure remains unchanged. Vasodilation results from the increase in peripheral oxygen consumption; the circulating blood volume also increases slightly.
RS   The thyroid hormones increase the rate and depth of respiration secondary to the increase in the basal metabolic rate.
CNS   The hormones have a stimulatory effect on central nervous system function; tremor and hyperreflexia may result. Their physiological function also includes mediation of negative feedback on the release of Thyroid Stimulating Hormone from the pituitary.

AS   Appetite is increased following the administration of thyroxine or triiodothyronine; the secretory activity and motility of the gastrointestinal tract are also increased.

GU   The thyroid hormones are involved in the control of sexual function and menstruation.

Metabolic/Other
Thyroid hormones promote gluconeogenesis and increase the mobilisation of glycogen stores. Lipolysis is stimulated leading to an increase in the concentration of free fatty acids; hypercholesterolaemia may result from increased cholesterol turnover. The rate of protein synthesis is enhanced.

Toxicity/Side Effects
Excessive administration of the thyroid hormones results in the clinical state of thyrotoxicosis.

Kinetics

Absorption   Both thyroxine and triiodothyronine are completely absorbed when administered orally.

Distribution   Both hormones are bound to thyroid-binding globulin and thyroid-binding pre-albumin in the plasma; thyroxine is 99.97% bound and triiodothyronine is 99.5% bound. The V_D of thyroxine is 0.2 l/kg and that of triiodothyronine is 0.5 l/kg.

Metabolism   35% of thyroxine is converted to triiodothyronine in the periphery (predominantly in the liver and kidney) and some to inactive reverse T3. Both thyroxine and triiodothyronine undergo conjugation to glucuronide and sulphate and are excreted in the bile; some enterohepatic circulation occurs.

Excretion   20–40% of an administered dose is excreted in the faeces unchanged. The clearance of thyroxine is 1.7 ml/min and the elimination half-life is 6–7 days; the clearance of triiodothyronine is 17 ml/min and the elimination half-life is 2 days.

Special Points   The thyroid hormones increase the anticoagulant activity of co-administered warfarin. Beta-adrenergic antagonists interfere with the conversion of thyroxine to triiodothyronine and lead to a relative increase in the inactive reverse T3 fraction.

Tolbutamide

Uses   Tolbutamide is used in the treatment of non-insulin-dependent (type II) diabetes mellitus.

Chemical   A sulphonylurea.

Presentation   As 500 mg tablets of tolbutamide.

Main Action   Hypoglycaemia.

Mode of Action   Tolbutamide acts by liberating insulin from pancreatic beta-cells; it appears to act by binding to the plasma membrane of the beta-cell and producing prolonged depolarisation, reducing the permeability of the membrane to potassium. This in turn leads to opening of calcium channels; the resulting influx of calcium causes triggering of insulin release. Sulphonylureas may also act by altering peripheral insulin-receptor number and sensitivity.

Route of Administration/Dose   The adult oral dose is 0.5–2 g daily.

Effects

Metabolic/Other   Tolbutamide causes a prompt and prolonged (6–12 hour) decrease in the blood sugar concentration; healthy subjects show a smaller decrease than do diabetic subjects. Sulphonylureas are ineffective in pancreatectomised patients and insulin-dependent diabetics. The drug also causes a decrease in the plasma free fatty acid concentration.

Toxicity/Side Effects   Occur in about 3% of patients who receive the drug. Gastrointestinal disturbances, cholestatic jaundice and alterations in liver function tests may occur. Tolbutamide has a disulfiram-like interaction when taken with alcohol. Rashes, reversible leucopenia, haemolytic anaemia and paraesthesiae have also been reported.

Kinetics

Absorption   The drug is 90% absorbed when administered orally; marked variations occur.

Distribution   Tolbutamide is 93% protein-bound in the plasma, predominantly to albumin; the V_D is 0.15 l/kg.

Metabolism   The drug is extensively metabolised in the liver by hydroxylation and carboxylation to active metabolites. There are genetically determined differences between individuals in the rate of metabolism.

Excretion   33% is excreted in the urine as the hydroxylated derivative; 66% as the carboxylated derivative. The clearance is 0.3 ml/min/kg and the elimination half-life is 7–10 hours.

Special Points It is generally recommended that oral hypoglycaemic agents are omitted on the morning of proposed surgery.

The drug should not be used in patients with hepatic or renal impairment. Tolbutamide is not removed by haemodialysis. An increase in cardiovascular mortality has been demonstrated in adults taking a fixed-dose regime of tolbutamide over a period of years.

The following drugs may potentiate the effect of sulphony-lureas either by displacement from plasma proteins or by inhibition of their hepatic metabolism and result in hypoglycaemia: NSAIDs, salicylates, sulphonamides, oral anticoagulants, MAOIs, and beta-adrenergic antagonists. Conversely, the following drugs tend to counteract the effect of sulphonylureas and result in loss of diabetic control: thiazide and other diuretics, steroids, phenothiazines, phenytoin, sympathomimetic agents and calcium antagonists.

Tramadol

Uses Tramadol is used in the management of moderate to severe pain.

Chemical A synthetic opioid of the aminocyclohexanol group. The drug is a racemic mixture of two enantiomers, (+) and (−) tramadol.

Presentation As a clear aqueous solution for injection containing 50 mg/ml and tablets containing 50/100/150/200/300/400 mg of tramadol hydrochloride.

Main Actions Centrally mediated analgesia.

Mode of Action Tramadol is a non-selective agonist at mu-, kappa- and delta-opioid receptors (with a higher relative affinity for mu-receptors). It also inhibits neuronal reuptake of noradrenaline and enhances serotonin (5-HT) release; inhibition of pain perception partly involves activation of descending serotonergic and noradrenergic pathways.

Routes of Administration/Doses Tramadol may be administered orally, intramuscularly or by slow intravenous injection or infusion. The adult dose is 50–100 mg 4–6-hourly for all routes of administration. The paediatric dose is 1–2 mg/kg 4–6 hourly.

Effects
CVS Tramadol has no clinically significant cardiovascular effects after intravenous administration.
RS Respiratory rate, minute volume and P_aCO_2 remain essentially unchanged following intravenous administration of therapeutic doses of the drug.
CNS Tramadol has an analgesic potency equivalent to pethidine. The analgesic effect is only partially (30%) reversed by naloxone.
AS Tramadol has no demonstrable effect on bile duct sphincter activity. Constipation occurs uncommonly.

Toxicity/Side Effects The principal side effects of tramadol are nausea, dizziness, sedation and diaphoresis. The potential for tolerance and dependence appear to be low.

Kinetics

Absorption The bioavailability following oral administration of the drug is 68–100%.

Distribution The drug is 20% protein-bound in the plasma; the V_D is 2.9–4.37 l/kg. 80% of an administered dose crosses the placenta.

Metabolism 85% of an administered dose is metabolised by demethylation in the liver. One metabolite (O-demethyl tramadol) is active.

Excretion 90% of the dose is excreted in the urine and 10% in the faeces. The clearance is 6.7–10.1 ml/kg/min and the elimination half-life is 270–450 minutes. The elimination half-life is doubled in patients with impaired renal or hepatic function.

Special Points The use of tramadol is not recommended in patients with end-stage renal failure; the dosage interval should be increased to 12 hours in patients with renal or hepatic impairment.

The drug is not licensed for intraoperative use as it may enhance intraoperative recall during enflurane/nitrous oxide anaesthesia.

Tramadol appears to be effective in the treatment of post-operative shivering.

The drug precipitates when mixed with diazepam or midazolam.

The drug is only slowly removed by haemodialysis or haemofiltration.

Tranexamic acid

Uses Tranexamic acid is used:
1. as a short-term adjunct to the management of haemorrhage due to increased fibrinolysis or fibrinogenolysis, e.g. post-prostatectomy bleeding, epistaxis or bleeding from cerebral aneurysms
2. prior to dental extraction in haemophiliacs
3. prior to repeat cardiac surgery
4. for the reversal of thrombolytic therapy and
5. in the chronic treatment of menorrhagia and
6. hereditary angioneurotic oedema.

Chemical Derivative of lysine.

Presentation A clear, colourless solution for intravenous use containing 100 mg/ml of tranexamic acid, in 500 mg tablet form and as a syrup containing 100 mg/ml.

Main Action Inhibition of fibrinolysis.

Mode of Action Tranexamic acid competitively inhibits the activation of plasminogen to plasmin.

Routes of Administration/Doses The intravenous dose is 15–25 mg/kg administered over 5 minutes. The corresponding oral dose is 1 g 6–8-hourly.

Effects
Metabolic/Other The thrombin time is increased; tranexamic acid has no effect on other coagulation parameters. Inhibition of complement pathways occurs following administration of the drug.

Toxicity/Side Effects Gastrointestinal disturbances may complicate the use of tranexamic acid.

Kinetics Data are incomplete.

Absorption Tranexamic acid is rapidly absorbed when administered orally; its bioavailability by this route is 34%.

Metabolism Little metabolism of tranexamic acid occurs.

Excretion 95% of an intravenously administered dose is excreted unchanged in the urine. The clearance is 1.6 ml/min/kg and elimination half-life is 1–2 hours.

Trichloroethylene

Uses Trichloroethylene is used:
1. for the induction and maintenance of general anaesthesia and has been used
2. for pain relief during labour.

Chemical A halogenated hydrocarbon.

Presentation As a blue liquid (that should be protected from light) that is coloured with waxoline blue to enable differentiation from chloroform. The commercial preparation contains 0.01% thymol which prevents decomposition on exposure to light; it is non-flammable in normal anaesthetic concentrations. The molecular weight of trichloroethylene is 131.4, the boiling point 67°C and the saturated vapour pressure is 8 kPa at 20°C. The MAC of trichloroethylene is 0.17, the oil/water solubility coefficient 400 and the blood/gas solubility coefficient 9.

Main Actions General anaesthesia (reversible loss of both awareness and recall of noxious stimuli) and analgesia.

Mode of Action The mechanism of general anaesthesia remains to be fully elucidated. General anaesthetics appear to disrupt synaptic transmission (especially in the area of the ventrobasal thalamus), predominantly by inhibiting neurotransmitter release and by interfering with the interaction of neurotransmitters with post-synaptic receptors. Their mode of action at the molecular level appears to involve expansion of hydrophobic regions in the neuronal membrane, either within the lipid phase or within hydrophobic sites in cell membrane proteins.

Route of Administration/Dose Trichloroethylene is administered by inhalation, conventionally via a calibrated vaporiser. The concentration used for the induction and maintenance of anaesthesia is 0.2–2%.

Effects
CVS Trichloroethylene is noted for its cardiovascular stability; the heart rate, blood pressure and cardiac output are little altered by the administration of the drug. Trichloroethylene has a marked propensity to cause dysrhythmias and sensitises the myocardium to the effects of circulating catecholamines.

RS The drug is moderately irritant to the respiratory tract and characteristically causes tachypnoea associated with a decreased tidal volume which may lead to both hypoxia and hypercapnia.

CNS The principal effect of trichloroethylene is general anaesthesia; the drug also has a marked analgesic effect. The drug increases cerebral blood flow, leading to an increase in intracranial pressure. A slight decrease in skeletal muscle tone results from the use of trichloroethylene.

AS Nausea and vomiting occur commonly with the use of the drug.

GU Trichloroethylene reduces the tone of the pregnant uterus when used in concentrations >0.5%.

Toxicity/Side Effects Trichloroethylene may provoke the appearance of myocardial dysrhythmias, particularly in the presence of hypoxia, hypercapnia or excessive catecholamine concentrations.

Kinetics

Absorption The major factors affecting the uptake of volatile anaesthetic agents are solubility, cardiac output and the concentration gradient between the alveoli and venous blood. Trichloroethylene is relatively soluble in blood; alveolar concentration therefore reaches inspired concentration relatively slowly, resulting in a slow induction of anaesthesia. An increase in the cardiac output increases the rate of alveolar uptake and slows the induction of anaesthesia. The concentration gradient between alveoli and venous blood approaches zero at equilibrium; a large concentration gradient favours the onset of anaesthesia.

Distribution The drug is initially distributed to organs with a high blood flow (the brain, heart, liver and kidney) and later to less well-perfused organs (muscles, fat and bone).

Metabolism 20% of an administered dose is metabolised in the liver to yield trichloroacetic acid, monochloroacetic acid and trichloroethanol (which is subsequently conjugated with glucuronide) and inorganic chloride.

Excretion 80% is exhaled unchanged; the metabolites are excreted in the urine over several days.

Special Points Trichloroethylene should not be used in a closed circuit with soda lime, since it decomposes in the presence of heat and alkali to form hydrochloric acid, carbon monoxide, dichloroacetylene and phosgene, all of which are toxic.

D-Tubocurarine

Uses Tubocurarine is used to facilitate intubation and controlled ventilation.

Chemical A monoquaternary alkaloid which is a derivative of isoquinoline.

Presentation As a clear, colourless solution for injection containing 10 mg/ml of tubocurarine chloride.

Main Action Competitive neuromuscular blockade.

Mode of Action Tubocurarine acts by competitive antagonism of acetylcholine at nicotinic (N2) receptors at the post-synaptic membrane of the neuromuscular junction; it also has some pre-junctional action.

Route of Administration/Dose Tubocurarine is administered intravenously; the normal intubating dose is 0.3–0.5 mg/kg with subsequent doses of one-third this amount. Satisfactory incubating conditions are produced within 3–5 minutes; a single dose lasts 20–30 minutes. The recovery index of the drug is 19–26 minutes.

Effects

CVS Hypotension and tachycardia may follow the administration of tubocurarine, resulting from the combined effects of histamine release, ganglion blockade and a decreased venous return caused by the loss of skeletal muscle tone. The drug appears to be concentrated in myocardial tissue and to protect against the development of cardiac dysrhythmias.

RS Neuromuscular blockade leads to apnoea. Tubocurarine has a marked potential for histamine release; bronchospasm is not uncommon. The drug also tends to increase bronchial secretions.

AS Tubocurarine increases salivation and decreases the tone and motility of the gastrointestinal tract.

Metabolic/Other The drug may cause decreased blood co-agulability as a result of the release of histamine from mast cells.

Toxicity/Side Effects Anaphylactoid reactions and profound hypotension may occur with the use of the drug. There are two reports of the development of malignant hyperpyrexia in patients who had received tubocurarine.

Kinetics

Absorption The drug is poorly and erratically absorbed after oral administration.

Distribution Tubocurarine is 42–58% protein-bound in the plasma, predominantly to albumin. The V_D is 0.19–0.41 l/kg. The drug does not cross the placental or blood–brain barrier.

Metabolism   Little metabolism of the drug occurs in man; 1% of the dose is demethylated in the liver.

Excretion   60–70% of an administered dose appears in the urine; the remainder is excreted in the bile. The clearance is 1.6–3 ml/min/kg and the elimination half-life is 0.9–3.1 hours. The drug is cumulative in the presence of renal impairment.

Special Points   The duration of action of tubocurarine, in common with other non-depolarising relaxants, is prolonged by hypokalaemia, hypocalcaemia, hypermagnesaemia, hypoproteinaemia, dehydration, acidosis and hypercapnia. The following drugs, when co-administered with non-depolarising relaxants, increase the effect of the latter: volatile and induction agents, fentanyl, suxamethonium, diuretics, calcium antagonists, alpha- and beta-adrenergic antagonists, protamine, metronidazole and the aminoglycoside antibiotics.

Neonates and infants have an increased sensitivity to tubocurarine, as determined by the plasma tubocurarine concentration at which 50% depression of EMG twitch height occurs. A decreased dose should not, however, be used in the very young, as the drug has a larger volume of distribution in this group. Additionally, the longer elimination half-life of the drug in neonates and infants carries the implication that the dose interval should be increased as the age of the patient decreases.

Vecuronium

Uses Vecuroniurn is used to facilitate intubation and controlled ventilation.

Chemical A bis-quaternary aminosteroid which is the mono-quaternary analogue of pancuronium.

Presentation As a lyophilised powder (containing a citrate phosphate buffer and mannitol) which is diluted in water prior to use to yield a clear, colourless solution containing 2 mg/ml of vecuronium bromide; the solution is stable for 24 hours.

Main Action Competitive neuromuscular blockade.

Mode of Action Vercuronium acts by competitive antagonism of aceylcholine at nicotinic (N2) receptors at the post-synaptic membrane of the neuromuscular junction; it also has some pre-junctional action.

Route of Administration/Dose Vecuronium is administered intravenously; the normal intubating dose is 0.08–0.1 mg/kg with subsequent doses of one-third this amount. The drug may also be infused at a rate of 50–80 µg/kg/hour. Satisfactory intubating conditions are produced within 2 minutes; there is a linear relationship between the dose and the duration of action. The recovery rate following administration by infusion is a similar to that observed after bolus administration; the recovery index is 14–30 minutes, according to dose. The drug is non-cumulative with repeated administration.

Effects
CVS Vecuronium has minimal cardiovascular effects; with large doses, a slight (9%) increase in cardiac output and (12%) decrease in systemic vascular resistance may occur. Unlike pancuronium, the drug does not antagonise fentanyl-induced bradycardia.
RS Neuromuscular blockade leads to apnoea. Vecuronium has a very low potential for histamine release; bronchospasm is extremely uncommon.
CNS The drug has no effect on intracranial or intraocular pressure.
AS Lower oesophageal sphincter pressure remains unaltered after the administration of vecuronium.
Metabolic/Other Vecuronium may decrease the partial thromboplastin time and prothrombin time.

Toxicity/Side Effects There have been rare reports of fatal anaphylactoid reactions with the administration of vecuronium. Cross-sensitivity may exist with rocuronium and pancuronium.

Kinetics

Distribution The drug is 60–90% protein-bound in the plasma; the V_D is 0.18–0.27 l/kg. The drug does not cross the placental or blood–brain barrier.

Metabolism Vecuronium is metabolised by deacetylation in the liver to the active metabolites 3- and 17-hydroxy and 3,17-dihydroxyvecuronium; they are present in very low concentrations and may be of clinical significance after prolonged dosing.

Excretion 25% of the dose is excreted unchanged in the urine and 20% unchanged in the bile; the clearance is 3–6.4 ml/kg/min and the elimination half-life is 31–80 minutes. Renal failure leads to a prolongation of the elimination half-life but to no clinically significant increase in the duration of action of vecuronium; hepatic failure causes a significant decrease in the clearance and consequent increase in the duration of action of the drug.

Special Points The duration of action of vecuronium, in common with other non-depolarising relaxants, is prolonged by hypokalaemia, hypocalcaemia, hypermagnesaemia, hypoproteinaemia, dehydration, acidosis and hypercapnia. The following drugs, when co-administered with non-depolarising relaxants, increase the effect of the latter: volatile and induction agents, fentanyl, suxamethonium, diuretics, calcium antagonists, alpha- and beta-adrenergic antagonists, protamine, metronidazole and the aminoglycoside antibiotics.

The use of vecuronium appears to be safe in patients susceptible to malignant hyperpyrexia.

Verapamil

Uses Verapamil is used in the treatment of:
1. hypertension of mild to moderate severity
2. angina and
3. paroxysmal supraventricular tachycardia, atrial fibrillation and flutter.

Chemical A synthetic papaverine derivative.

Presentation As 40/80/120/160/180/240 mg tablets and as a clear solution for injection of a racemic mixture of verapamil hydrochloride containing 2.5 mg/ml.

Main Actions Antihypertensive and antianginal.

Mode of Action Verapamil causes competitive blockade of cell membrane slow calcium ion channels leading to a decreased influx of calcium ions into vascular smooth muscle and myocardial cells. This results in electromechanical decoupling, inhibition of contraction and relaxation of cardiac and smooth muscle fibres leading to coronary and systemic arterial vasodilation.

Routes of Administration/Doses The adult oral dose is 240–480 mg daily in 2–3 divided doses. The corresponding intravenous dose in 5–10 mg administered over 30 seconds; the injection should cease as soon as the desired effect is achieved. The peak effect after intravenous administration occurs at 3–5 minutes and the duration of action is 10–20 minutes.

Effects
CVS Verapamil is a class IV antiarrhythmic agent; it decreases automaticity and conduction velocity and increases the refractory period. Atrio-ventricular conduction is slowed; the drug appears to be taken, up and bound specifically by atrio-ventricular nodal tissue. The drug causes a decrease in the systemic vascular resistance and is a potent coronary artery vasodilator. Verapamil has negative dromotropic and inotropic effects which are enhanced by acidosis.
CNS Cerebral vasodilation occurs after the administration of verapamil. The drug has local anaesthetic properties.
GU Verapamil decreases renovascular resistance.

Toxicity/Side Effects Oral administration of the drug may lead to dizziness, flushing, nausea and first- or second-degree heart block. Intravenous administration may precipitate heart failure in patients with impaired left ventricular function and precipitate ventricular tachycardia or fibrillation in patients with the Wolff-Parkinson-White syndrome.

Kinetics

Absorption Verapamil is, completely absorbed when administered orally; the bioavailability is 10–22% due to a significant first-pass metabolism.

Distribution The drug is 90% protein-bound in the plasma; the V_D is 3.1–4.9 l/kg.

Metabolism Occurs by demethylation and dealkylation in the liver – the metabolites possess some activity.

Excretion 70% of the dose is excreted in the urine and 16% in the faeces. The clearance is 6.8–16.8 ml/min/kg and the elimination half-life is 3–7 hours. The dose should be reduced in patients with significant hepatic impairment.

Special Points The effects of volatile agents and beta-adrenergic antagonists on myocardial contractility and conduction are synergistic with those of verapamil; caution should be exercised when these combinations are used. The drug increases the serum concentrations of co-administered digoxin.

Verapamil and dantrolene administered concurrently in animals cause hyperkalaemia leading to ventricular fibrillation; these drugs are not recommended for use together in man. The drug decreases the MAC of halothane in animal models; chronic exposure to the drug may potentiate the actions of both depolarising and non-depolarising relaxants. Verapamil attenuates the pressor response to laryngoscopy and intubation.

Verapamil is not removed by haemodialysis.

Warfarin

Uses   Warfarin is used:
1. in the prophylaxis of systemic embolisation in patients with rheumatic heart disease and atrial fibrillation and in patients with prosthetic heart valves and
2. in the prophylaxis and treatment of deep vein thrombosis and pulmonary embolism.

Chemical   A synthetic coumarin derivative.

Presentation   As tablets containing 0.5/1/3/5 mg of a racemic mixture of warfarin sodium.

Main Action   Anticoagulation.

Mode of Action   Warfarin prevents the synthesis of the vitamin K-dependent clotting factors (II, VII, IX and X) in the liver. The formation of fully active clotting factors is dependent on the carboxylation of their precursor proteins; during this reaction vitamin K is oxidised to vitamin K 2,3-epoxide; warfarin prevents the reduction of this episode back to vitamin K. This results in vitamin K depletion and a decrease in the rate of formation of complete clotting factors. The S enantiomer is 2–5 times more potent than the R enantiomer.

Route of Administration/Dose   The adult oral dose is usually 3–9 mg/day, according to response as measured by the prothrombin time. The maximum anticoagulant effect occurs 18–72 hours after the administration of a loading dose.

Effects   Warfarin has no clinically significant effects other than its anticoagulant effect.

Toxicity/Side Effects   Haemorrhage is the most frequent side effect. Hypersensitivity reactions and gastrointestinal upsets may occur. The drug appears to be teratogenic if taken during pregnancy.

Kinetics

Absorption   The drug is rapidly and completely absorbed from the stomach and upper gastrointestinal tract and has an oral bioavailability of 100%.

Distribution   Warfarin is 99% protein-bound in the serum, predominantly to albumin. The V_D is 0.1–0.16 l/kg.

Metabolism   Warfarin is virtually completely metabolised in the liver by oxidation (of the L-form) and reduction (of the D-form); these metabolites are then conjugated with glucuronide.

Excretion   The metabolites are excreted in the faeces and urine. The clearance is 3.26–3.8 ml/min/kg and the elimination half-life of warfarin ranges from 35 to 45 hours; this is decreased in patients with renal impairment.

Special Points   The response to warfarin treatment is monitored in the laboratory by the one-stage prothrombin time, which is particularly sensitive to the activity of factors II, VII and X. The INR should be maintained at 2–4.5 times the control value. Many factors may affect warfarin control; in particular, the drug may exhibit significant interactions with many other drugs. The activity of warfarin may be potentiated by alcohol, amiodarone, cimetidine, sulphonamides, salicylates and other NSAIDs and many antibiotics, including co-trimoxazole, erythromycin, chloramphenicol, metronidazole and tetracyclines. The activity of warfarin may be decreased by many drugs, including barbiturates, the oral contraceptive pill and carbamazipine.

Control of anticoagulation in the peri-operative period requires special attention. This is usually achieved by transferring the patient to heparin prior to and immediately after surgery; the INR should ideally be less than 2 for routine surgery. Acute reversal of the effects of warfarin can be achieved by the administration of fresh frozen plasma. Alternatively, 1 mg of vitamin K will reverse its effects within 12 hours and 10 mg will prevent re-warfarinisation due to the saturation of liver stores.

Spinal and epidural anaesthesia are contraindicated in patients anticoagulated with warfarin.

Zidovudine

Uses Zidovudine is used to reduce the incidence of neoplasia and opportunistic infections in patients with the acquired immunodeficiency syndrome (AIDS) or AIDS-related complex (ARC).

Chemical A thymidine analogue.

Presentation As capsules containing 100/250/300 mg, a syrup containing 10 mg/ml of zidorudine and as intravenous solution 10 mg/ml which needs dilution prior to infusion.

Main Action Antiviral.

Mode of Action The drug is initially phosphorylated to an active form which becomes incorporated into intracellular viral DNA by acting as a substrate for, and inhibitor of, viral reverse transcriptase. It thereby prevents the uptake of thymidine into viral DNA. Once incorporated, it terminates the viral DNA chain.

Route of Administration/Doses The adult oral dose is 200–300 mg (3.5 mg/kg) 4-hourly; the dosage interval should be increased to 8 hours if the haemoglobin level decreases or neutropenia occurs and the drug should be discontinued if the haemoglobin falls to below 7.5 g/dl or the neutrophil count falls to less than 0.75×10^9/litre.

Effects
Metabolic/Other The use of zidovudine is associated with significant weight gain, increased well-being and improved survival rates in patients with AIDS or ARC. The drug produces a decrease in the incidence of opportunistic infections and an increased tendency to clear these when they do occur. Zidovudine appears to slow the rate of neurological deterioration in this group of patients.

Toxicity/Side Effects Severe haematological disturbances (anaemia, leucopenia and neutropenia) occur in 45% of patients receiving zidovudine. Headache; nausea, insomnia and myalgia occur more commonly than in patients receiving placebo.

Kinetics

Absorption The drug is well absorbed with an oral bioavailability of 60–70%.

Distribution Zidovudine is 34–38% protein-bound in the plasma; the V_D is 1.4 l/kg.

Metabolism Occurs in the liver by glucuronidation.

Excretion 10–20% appears unchanged in the urine, the remainder is excreted by renal tubular secretion as the glucuronide metabolite. The clearance is 21.67 ml/min/kg and the elimination half-life is 1–1.5 hours.

Special Points   There is a theoretical risk of an interaction between nitrous oxide and zidovudine, since both may cause decreased availability of thymidine-5-triphosphate for DNA synthesis.

Accumulation of the drug is likely (although unproven) in patients with renal or hepatic impairment.

The combination of acyclovir and zidovudine appears to increase significantly long-term survival in patients with AIDS or ARC.

Index of drug derivation

Index of drug derivation

Index of medical uses